DIFFICULT ORTHOPEDIC DIAGNOSIS

DIFFICULT
ORTHOPEDIC
DIAGNOSIS

By

LEWIS COZEN, M.D.

Attending Surgeon, L. A. Orthopedic Hospital
Senior Attending Physician, Cedars of Lebanon Hospital
Associate Clinical Professor, UCLA Medical School
Senior Attending Surgeon, Wadsworth General Hospital
Los Angeles, California

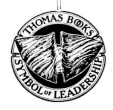

CHARLES C THOMAS · PUBLISHER
Springfield · *Illinois* · *U.S.A.*

Published and Distributed Throughout the World by
CHARLES C THOMAS • PUBLISHER
BANNERSTONE HOUSE
301-327 East Lawrence Avenue, Springfield, Illinois, U.S.A.
NATCHEZ PLANTATION HOUSE
735 North Atlantic Boulevard, Fort Lauderdale, Florida, U.S.A.

© *1972, by* CHARLES C THOMAS • PUBLISHER

ISBN 0-398-02212-7

Library of Congress Catalog Card Number: 74-172452

With THOMAS BOOKS *careful attention is given to all details of
manufacturing and design. It is the Publisher's desire to present books
that are satisfactory as to their physical qualities and artistic possibilities
and appropriate for their particular use.* THOMAS BOOKS *will be true
to those laws of quality that assure a good name and good will.*

Printed in the United States of America

HH-11

To
Paul R. McMaster
and
Charles L. Lowman
Masters of Clinical Observation

PREFACE

The purpose of this monograph is to describe some of the difficult diagnostic problems that are encountered in an orthopedic practice. Any experienced orthopedic surgeon should be able to write a treatise of this type and it would be different in each case depending upon the experience of the orthopedist. This small book is based largely on my experience for the past thirty years.

The work is not encyclopedic. Not included are many rare diseases of the musculoskelectal system. Most of the common diseases are omitted if they present no real diagnostic difficulty. Omitted are those rare and perhaps interesting anomalies and diseases that are not especially significant as far as making a serious difference in the patient's welfare if the diagnosis is made correctly or not. I have tried to emphasize the diseases and other conditions that might jeopardize the patient's course or influence the family's decision in regard to prognosis. I am sure I have neglected some important clinical entities in that regard and therefore the book is incomplete. Perhaps some readers will be kind enough to call my attention to areas that I have overlooked. Should I then in a subsequent edition have a chapter on overlooked difficult orthopedic diagnosis?

Dr. Win Kulik, associate radiologist of the Othopedic Hospital, Los Angeles, was kind enough to give me the x-ray films that are used for the illustrations. I am indebted to him.

LEWIS COZEN, M.D.

CONTENTS

DIFFICULT ORTHOPEDIC DIAGNOSIS

THE FOOT

Tarsal Tunnel Syndrome

Pain of a vague nature in the foot can be caused by the tarsal tunnel syndrome. The pain is vague, and it can be present anywhere in the toes or in the arch of the foot or on either side of the foot. The pain that is present is not constant, and it is not always relieved by bed rest.

Abnormal physical findings are few. There may be some hypesthesia to touch and pin prick, especially over the medial aspect of the foot and over the great toe area, but even this may be absent. The diagnosis is made by eliciting abnormal conduction time of the posterior tibial nerve at the ankle area. Conduction time studies are made of the posterior tibial nerve, and a delay in the conduction time, if present, is localized in the malleolar lesion of the ankle. Rarely the syndrome is accompanied by tenosynovitis of the posterior tibial tendon, and in such an instance there will be some swelling and tenderness posterior to the medial malleolus. If posterior tibial tenosynovitis is indeed present, injection of the tendon sheath with a small quantity of Hydrocortone® will give relief of the pain. Such relief will in addition help make the diagnosis more certain. An inner wedge or raise of the heel to relieve some tension of the posterior tibial nerve may be tried also. This correction may also aid in the diagnosis, since relief of the vague pain would be one indication of pressure on the posterior tibial nerve. In large measure, however, the treatment is surgical with exposure of the posterior tibial nerve behind the medial malleolus and sectioning of the retinaculum covering the nerve here.

Dupuytren's Contracture

Dupuytren's contracture of the foot is not common but is of some importance. Its importance stems from the fact that it can be one of the somewhat unusual causes of pain in the foot, and

3

secondly, it can be treated erroneously if it is not diagnosed correctly. If the diagnosis is not made, it is unlikely that the correct treatment, which is complete excision of the entire plantar fascia, would be done. If it is mistakenly thought to be a small ganglion or nodule in the foot and the local small mass is removed, the painful tumor will almost inevitably recur and often the patient has more pain and there is also increased size of the nodule in the plantar fascia.

The plantar fascia of Dupuytren's contracture is tender and often there is a slight nodular enlargement in the area of involvement. Usually the tender nodule is in the center of the plantar aspect of the foot and it is felt directly under the skin. There may or may not be contracture with fascitis of the palmar fascia of either one or both hands. There may also be involvement of the penis with contracture of the fibrous tissue there, and then it would be called Peyronie's disease. It is of course possible that the nodular enlargement of the bottom of the foot may be caused by other conditions, such as malignant synovioma, fibrosarcoma, or foreign body granulomas. X-ray films of the foot must be made in order to make sure that there is not a needle that has been embedded in some of the granulomatous tissue within the foot, or that the tender mass on the bottom of the foot is not an extension of an abscess from the tarsal bones. Examination of the popliteal and the inguinal glands would disclose no adenopathy there if the condition is indeed Dupuytren's contracture of the foot.

The patient is told of the probably diagnosis, and to verify the diagnosis an incision must be made over the plantar fascia. If the nodule is seen to be within the fascia, the incision must be lengthened to the entire extent of the plantar fascia and the fascia must be completely excised as previously noted.

Fatigue Fractures

Fatigue fractures of the foot can be, and often are, very deceptive in diagnosis. One thinks of the fatigue fracture as occurring in soldiers or in other young men who march without adequate training for long periods. Young men are not the only ones who have fatigue fractures. Old people, especially if they are obese and if the bones of their feet become osteoporotic, can fracture one or more metatarsals simply by going shopping two or three times a week in the large supermarkets. Fractured metatarsal can occur in women if they must walk on heavily carpeted floors frequently during the day.

Where there is some generalized diseases that makes bone atrophic, fatigue fractures can occur. This is especially true in rheumatoid arthritis, where there may be one or more ankylosed joints on the affected leg increasing the stress on the bone with each step.

In young people participating in sports, fatigue fractures are common and are easily overlooked in any bone, not only in the metatarsal. The fractures can occur in any bone of the lower extremity, from the metatarsals to and including the pelvis. The fatigue fracture can take place in children five years of age, as well as in teenagers and in the aged. The vague pains that some boys or girls have and are called growing pains are at times caused by fatigue fractures.

To make certain of the diagnosis, the fracture must be seen on the x-ray film. Clinically, if the bone that is involved is superficial, as in a metatarsal bone, there is some swelling and tenderness. If the femur is involved, clinical signs can be completely absent.

Repeated x-ray films must be made if pain persists in anyone suspected of a march fracture to find the telltale periosteal proliferation of a fatigue fracture. Laminograms can be helpful if the x-ray film on repeated occasions is normal and the diagnosis is still suspected.

It is important to assure the diagnosis is march fracture since it is so easily confused with other conditions, such as neurosis, arthritis, and osteosarcoma.

Anterior Tibial Syndrome

The anterior tibial syndrome is a cause for misdiagnosis at times. The syndrome usually takes place following severe trauma to the proximal portion of the lower leg, often when a comminuted fracture of the tibia and fibula are present here. If the trauma is severe enough, there need not be a fracture, however;

the acute form of the syndrome can also occur as it was first described after a marching incident. The syndrome consists of necrosis of the muscles on the anterior portion of the lower leg as a result of impairment of their blood supply. This form of partial necrosis of the leg can take place in the presence of patent arteries to the leg so that the physician is misled by noting a vigorous anterior and posterior tibial pulse at the ankle.

There is inordinate pain accompanying the anterior tibial syndrome, and this is probably the most important clue to diagnosis. There is also moderate to marked swelling present, and swelling can be noted at the proximal end of the toes distal to the plaster of paris cast which is usually applied for this fracture. The patient when asked to do so will be unable to move his toes and the examining physician will then think that he has a peroneal nerve palsy. Indeed paralysis of the peroneal nerve and anterior tibial syndrome often accompany each other. There is numbness and hypesthesia of the toes usually present but color and temperature of the toes is normal, and this finding, along with palpable pulses at the ankle, negate the diagnosis of impending gangrene of the entire leg. Other compartments of the lower leg including the posterior compartment may become involved.

Once the diagnosis is suspected, the cast and any other circumferential bandages must be removed. The extent of the edema and induration on the anterior portion of the lower leg is noted, and if there is any doubt concerning patency of the anterior and posterior tibial arteries an arteriogram is performed. If the arteriogram reveals the arteries to be indeed patent, incision of the skin and fascia on the anterior aspect of the lower leg must be performed at once. If the arteries are occluded, then arterial reconstruction must be performed.

The chronic form of the anterior tibial syndrome can take place in people who march excessively and complain of vague pain in the lower leg. This is entirely different and is merely a painful affection without any danger to the muscles or any other structure of the lower leg. There is usually tenderness over the anterior tibial and extensor muscles as they originate on the anterior surface of the lower leg.

If there is crepitus noted when the patient moves his toes or ankle, then a diagnosis of chronic tendinitis is made and this may be present with the chronic form of anterior tibial syndrome.

Although it is not proposed here to deal in detail with treatment, the course of treatment consists here of resting the part, elevation, and at times local injections of cortisone.

Juvenile Planter Fascitis

An uncommon cause of pain in the foot, this has been shown to cause pain on the plantar aspect of the foot in children. The diagnosis can only be made on biopsy and the pathologist who reviews the sections must be well versed in this condition, for it is a rare one and some pathologists have never encountered it. It is important to differentiate this affection from fibrosarcoma or synovioma although the affection is a persistent and recurring one and often the patient must undergo frequent excisions of the plantar fascia before cure is obtained.

Bone Tumors

Bone tumors of various types affect the bones of the foot, but the diagnosis of bone tumor is often missed because they occur most frequently in the long bones rather than in the foot. For instance, Ewing's tumor can have its onset manifested by vague pain in the heel or other area, and even when the x-ray film reveals a radiolucent area within the calcaneus, it is easily passed over as an innocuous local infection. Osteoid osteomas also have been found in the bones of the foot. The youngster who complains of pain in the foot that is relieved by aspirin should be suspected of having an osteoid osteoma. Careful search by good x-ray films must be made since the lesion may be tiny and may be mistaken for a variation of the growth pattern of one of the bones of the foot. It is therefore wise here as in other bone conditions in children to have films of the opposite foot made for comparison.

It is worth repeating that almost all bone tumors can develop in the various bones of the foot, and their existence must be recognized in any patient, young or old, who complains of pain here.

Granulomas

Granulomas such as tuberculosis, though rare, can and do occasionally occur in the tarsal joints, ankle joint, or metatarsalphalangeal joint. There is swelling, low-grade fever, and night pain. The x-ray films reveal bone demineralization with invasion and destruction of the affected joint. The history of exposure to a tuberculous patient may be obtained. Tuberculin test is usually positive, and a chest film may disclose evidence of tuberculosis. This is another condition whose diagnosis is missed at times because of its infrequency today.

Other granulomata such as coccidioidomycosis may also manifest themselves in the foot region. The history of vague pain and the clinical findings of swelling and tenderness similar to the findings present in a patient with tuberculosis of the foot make one aware of that possibility in a patient who has been in an area where the disease is endemic. These areas are the San Joaquin Valley of California, Arizona, and Mexico. The roentgen appearance is similar to that of tuberculosis, and diagnosis must be suspected so that the physician may order a coccidioidomycosis skin test or a serum antibody test. Biopsy will reval the spherules characteristic of this fungus.

Other fungal diseases can affect the foot—blastomycosis, Madura foot, actinomycosis—and these conditions produce symptoms and physical signs similar to the other granulomata. Their diagnosis is made usually only after a biopsy has been performed. Brodie's abscess (chronic osteomyelitis) will cause symptoms and signs similar to the granulomata.

Intermittent Claudication

The cause of pain in the foot may be intermittent claudication caused by inadequate arterial supply to the foot. The patient may complain of vague pain in the foot, the pain being increased on walking and relieved by rest. Do not be misled by the presence of palpable pulsations at the ankle. The pulsations may decrease and disappear after some exercise, indicating the inadequacy of blood supply when the foot and leg are exercised. There should be some evidence of impaired blood supply to the foot, such as absence of any hair on the foot, abnormal color of the foot, blanching of the foot on elevation, and prolonged filling of the veins when the foot is held in a dependent position. The patient should be asked to walk back and forth in the office for a few minutes until he states that the pain which bothers him has recurred. The patient is examined at that time to see if the pulses which were present before he started walking are absent now. Thus the diagnosis of insufficient blood supply to the foot is confirmed and he is sent to a vascular surgeon, who will perform an anteriogram.

Dislocations of the Tarsal Joints

Dislocations of the tarsal joints are missed occasionally. After an injury has been sustained, the tarsometatarsal joint can be partially dislocated, and if a straight anteroposterior and a straight lateral view are not made, a partial dislocation of the tarsometatarsal joint can be easily missed. Other x-ray views can be made if one is suspicious of a subluxation here, and one should order comparable films of the opposite foot if there is some doubt as to the presence or absence of a dislocation.

Dislocation of the interphalangeal joints of the toe is another dislocation that is easily missed. It is difficult to get a good lateral view of an injured toe, and the injured toe should be examined radiologically in this position if one is suspicious. The anteroposterior view of the toe gives some clue to the diagnosis of dislocation, since the joint space of the interphalangeal joint appears to be narrowed. In such an instance, the x-ray technician should be asked to separate the toes and to take a straight lateral view of the individual toe instead of the usual overlapping or oblique views.

Fractures of the Tarsal Bones

Fractures of the tarsal bones can be missed occasionally. This is particularly true of the anterior lip of the calcaneus (Gelman fracture) and also of the body of the calcaneus itself. Again, by having satisfactory films in the straight lateral and the AP views, one will be less apt to miss the slight indications of these fractures.

Rheumatoid Arthritis

Rheumatoid arthritis can manifest itself in the foot and may cause pain in the foot of a young or old person. The pain may be accompanied by very little in the way of objective findings.

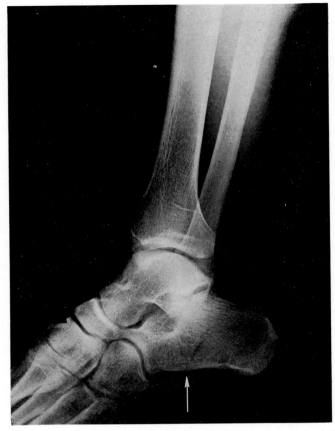

Figure 1. Fracture of the calcaneus. An excellent quality of the x-ray film and careful scrutiny are necessary to show the slight crack in the calcaneus. If the diagnosis is missed, unprotected weight-bearing may cause severe displacement of such a fracture. Incidentally, in this case there is also a calcaneal navicular congenital synostosis.

It becomes necessary therefore to suspect the presence of rheumatoid arthritis in the foot of either a child or an adult who complains of pain in one foot where there is no very defenite cause for the pain; in other words, where there is no history of a severe injury. On examination, there may be slight tenderness and may or may not be some swelling of the involved joint area. Characteristically the sedimentation rate is elevated, but in children the latex test for rheumatoid arthritis is usually nagative whereas in the adult it is more likely to be positive. It is wise where the diagnosis of rheumatoid arthritis is suspected, therefore, to start a program of conservative therapy including the use of salicylates. Salicylate medication orally may aid the pain and will give the physician time to observe the patient's progress. Thus other diseases, such as tarsal tunnel syndrome or tumors of the foot or granulomas such as tuberculosis, will become manifest by the peculiarities of each such disease. The x-ray findings in rheumatoid arthritis early are either absent or so nonspecific that the diagnosis is not helped. Of course if there is the telltale atrophy of the bone with the early erosion of joint surface, the diagnosis is made more secure.

Lupus Erythematosus

L.E., or lupus erythematosus, is an affection that is also rather easily missed because the early findings of lupus erythematosus may be mild joint pain and the pain is also similar to that of rheumatoid arthritis. It may be some time before the kidney involvement, the cardiac involvement, and the findings of the L.E. cells in the blood smear make the presence of this disease evident.

Subungual Exostosis

Subungual exostosis is a minor affection of the toe, but it can create pain in the toe. The tip of the toe is painful and there is tenderness on pressure over the toenail. In such cases a lateral x-ray film of the toe will disclose a spur projecting from the bony distal phalanx pressing under the nail.

Glomus Tumors

Glomus tumors of the toes or foot are also missed frequently. These are rare small angiomatous tumors usually located under the toenail area. They can occur, however, in any area of the foot or, for that matter, anyplace else. There is point tenderness over the small tumor. When the growth is present under the toenail, often it is identified by the bluish-black color. The color can become more pronounced if the examiner applies an ice bag to the toe or has the patient soak his foot in cold water.

Myositis Ossificans Progressiva

Myositis ossificans progressiva, peculiarly enough, can be diagnosed in a child often by the shortness of the first metatarsal and the first toe. In a youngster where there is new bone formation in one of the extremities or in the upper part of the back, an x-ray film of the foot that reveals an abnormally short first metatarsal should make the physician aware of the possibility of myositis ossificans progressiva. Of course this will alter his prognosis from that of a benign local process to a lethal generalized disease.

Van Creveld Syndrome

The Van Creveld syndrome is a congenital affection of the toes wherein there is syndactilism of the toes associated with congenital heart disease. Where syndactilism or other malformations of the toes is noted, examination of the heart is indicated to see if this syndrome is indeed present.

Congenital Vertical Talus

Flatfoot in the infant can be confusing. Because congenital vertical talus should be treated differently from the relaxed flatfoot, the distinction is important. In the flatfoot caused by vertical talus, the sole of the foot is in a rocker shape. The heel will, on close inspection, be found to be drawn proximally in a position of equinus. An x-ray film of the foot, especially a standing film, will disclose vertical position of the talus with dorsiflexion of the metatarsals and with equinus position of the calcaneus.

Tarsal Coalition (Rigid Flatfoot)

Flat feet of the usual type in both the youngster and in the adult should not be confused with the type that is caused by tarsal coalition. The prognosis and treatment for the tarsal coalition type of flatfoot is quite different from that of the usual flexible flatfoot. In the tarsal coalition patients there is limitation of inversion and eversion whereas this motion is perfectly free in the flexible type of flatfoot. Special x-ray films including oblique views of the tarsus and the Harris view, which is a tangential longitudinal x-ray view of the medial aspect of the tarsal bones, reveal incomplete or complete synostosis between some of the tarsal bones. The most common anomaly of this type is the calcaneal navicular bar. The less frequent talocalcaneal coalition is to be found by the Harris view previously noted.

THE LEG

Intervertebral Disc Lesions

Intervertebral disc lesions can cause pain only in the foot or leg. It is therefore important to recognize this fact and to give credence to the possibility of pain in the leg and even in the lower leg and foot having its origin from an intervertebral disc lesion with nerve root pressure in the lower part of the spine. One usually assumes there will be back pain and hip pain with disc lesions, but this is not always the case. Therefore, in any patient who complains of lower leg or foot pain for which no other more obvious cause is found, examination both clinically and radiologically of the lumbar spine must be made. Neurological examination must be performed as well, and even the most subtle changes and abnormalities may be noted. For instance, there may be only slight limitation of straight leg raising and there may be minimal weakness of the calf muscles found in the examination. Of course if there are such obvious findings as pain and some limitation of motion of the lumbar spine, the diagnosis of a radicular syndrome becomes easier.

Spinal Cord Tumors

Spinal cord tumors may cause the same type of pain distal to the spine. In other words, pain may be present only in the foot or lower leg in the presence of a spinal cord tumor. The typical findings characterizing the presence of a spinal cord tumor also may be minimal. If the pain in the foot and lower leg is present at night while at rest, this could be significant of a spinal cord tumor. Of course if there has been a past history of a malignancy, one is more prone to suspect a metastatic lesion. X-ray films of the spine as well as of the pelvis must not only be seen, but they must be repeated frequently if the pain persists and if there is any reason whatsoever to suspect the presence of a cord tumor. Within a matter of a week, destructive changes of bone can be visible where none were present in the x-ray films a week earlier. Of course such additional studies as elevated alkaline phosphatase and calcium, and an elevated sedimentation rate can also be indicative. A radioactive strontium bone scan will also be very helpful.

Bone Tumors

Bone tumors of various types can cause pain in the lower leg. When there is pain *at night* either in a child or in an adult, and the pain is located or localized in the lower leg, one should be particularly suspicious of the presence of a bone tumor and more especially of malignant bone tumor. Malignant bone tumors are osteosarcoma, Ewing's tumor, fibrosarcoma, rare primary tumors, and metastatic tumors of bone. The latter, namely the metastatic tumors of bone, are more common in the proximal end of the tibia but they can be in any bone in the body.

Malignant bone tumors do not necessarily cause severe pain. The pain may be deceptive. It may be minimal and even intermittent. In other words, one must not be deceived by the atypical type of pain that is present. Repeated examination and repeated x-ray examinations are necessary when the pain in a leg continues and no definite cause for it is found. X-ray changes may be minimal or may be absent at first. For instance, multiple myeloma often is identified by radiolucency or osteoporosis rather than by any destructive appearance seen on the x-ray films. Changes in the serum proteins in myeloma plus the increased sedimentation rate and the abnormal urinary findings are to be looked for.

BENIGN TUMORS OF THE TIBIA AND FIBULA. Benign tumors of the tibia and fibula are the osteoid osteoma, aneurysmal bone cyst, unicameral bone syst, chondromyxoid fibroma, periosteal chondroma, as well as others. In the history, osteoid osteoma of course has the typical story of relief from pain by aspirin. The pain of the other benign tumors is usually not severe and is intermittent in type.

GIANT CELL TUMOR. Giant cell tumor of bone is classified separately since it at times is benign and at times malignant. In all of these bone tumors, there is an x-ray appearance that is present more or less consistently with each more than with any other type of tumor, but ultimately the diagnosis must be made by biopsy of the bone. Even here one must accept the fact that several repeated biopsies at different intervals may be necessary to make the diagnosis. In other words, if the diagnosis seems to be unclear because of recurrence of the tumor or because of the pathologist's inability to make a definite diagnosis, the biopsy must be repeated. One should try to have the biopsy material from the edge of the tumor if at all possible.

ADAMANTINOMA. One unique tumor is the adamantinoma. This peculiar tumor apparently derives from the endothelial cells of the blood vessels and occurs in the tibia. It is a rare and a locally malignant tumor. Diagnosis is made almost invariably by biopsy of the destructive area of the tibia.

Fibrosarcoma

Fibrosarcoma is a malignant tumor that can occur in the bone or in the soft tissues. In this category reticulum cell sarcoma must be mentioned. I do not believe it is necessary to identify the peculiarities of each one of these tumors since they are easily handled in most textbooks. I refer to both the radiologic and the histologic appearance of these various tumors.

Tumors of the Soft Tissues of the Lower Leg—Benigin and Malignant

Of course the malignant tumors of the muscle and fibrous tissue and even the skin usually cause more pain than do benign tumors. The rhabdosarcoma, the lymphosarcoma, and the fibrosarcoma of the calf or other soft tissue will usually cause aching during the night. A benign tumor, such as a fibroma of the soft tissue, is unlikely to cause pain.

HEMANGIOMA OF THE CALF. This is a tumor that causes pain of a very indefinite and elusive type. Although it is not a common one, it is usually not diagnosed because of the difficulty of making the diagnosis. It occurs more commonly in children than in adults, and the pain is usually in the proximal half just distal to the knee joint. These children, because of the vagueness of the pain, are often labeled as being neurotic. There is one physical finding that is almost universally present, and that is tenderness in the region of the tumor. The tenderness must be elicited by deep palpation since the tumor is usually deep in the calf rather than being directly on the tibia. The hemangioma is often small. In such a patient an arteriogram may be helpful, or it may be necessary to perform direct surgical exploration of the area with an effective tourniquet to visualize the small mass of bool vessels that are present.

Peroneal Palsy

Peroneal palsy or foot drop is an affection that can easily be overlooked. The patient who has back pain because of a lumbosacral disc syndrome can be examined many times and the presence of foot drop may not be noted unless it is looked for specifically. In other words, at the time of each examination of the patient with back pain, the strength of the extensors and flexors of the foot must be tested to see if weakness of some of the muscles of the foot resulting in partial foot drop is present. The patient himself is often unaware of the weakness since he interprets any slight difficulty in walking that he may have as a result of his pain.

There are many causes for peroneal palsy, some of which are elusive. Some people who keep their legs crossed for long periods of time, for instance when viewing television, will develop foot drop as a result of pressure on the peroneal nerve over the head of the fibula. Other causes are alcoholism, malnutrition, lead poisoning, lues, and spinal cord tumor. One cause that is not thought of commonly is a ganglion in the region of the head of the fibula. Other tumors, benign or malignant, may cause pressure over the peroneal nerve, and of course these are usually felt on examination or their pressure is seen on x-ray films.

After a fracture of the tibia or fibula there may be peroneal palsy as a result of hemorrhage surrounding the peroneal nerve as it winds around the head of the fibula, and this should be thought of in every case of a fracture of the lower leg so that strength of the toe extensors should be examined periodically.

Psoas Abscess

Abscess of the psoas muscle is indeed a difficult diagnosis to make. It is especially difficult if the abscess takes place as a result of hematogenous infection without any involvement of the dorsal or lumbar spine. The usual cause of psoas abscesses is tuberculosis of the spine. Even here, evidence of osteomyelitis or of tuberculous infection of the bone can be delayed, and the presence of the psoas abscess will be the first indication of bone involvement of the spine.

The first indication of psoas abscess is usually vague pain in the leg. The pain is usually in the femoral area and is caused by pressure on the lumbar nerve plexus by the enlarging abscess of the psoas muscle. There is usually a spiking type of fever if the abscess is nontuberculous, the fever commencing at about the time that the vague pain starts. Somewhat later there is some tenderness and swelling in the upper thigh region. It must be remembered that if the psoas abscess tracks all the way down into the lesser trochanter of the femur where the psoas muscle inserts, the pus can then burrow under the fascia to the knee.

There may be vague mild pain in the lower spine even if there

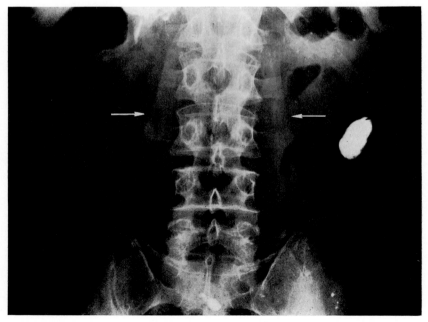

Figure 2A.   Psoas shadows equal on both right and left sides in a 60-year-old male three years before symptoms.

is no bone involvement accompanying the abscess in the muscle. Motion of the spine will also be normal and there will be no spine tenderness and no paravertebral tenderness even with the presence of a large psoas abscess. Of course if the spine is involved there will be tenderness of the spine as noted in another section where osteomyelitis of the spine has been mentioned.

There may be slight limitation of rotation of the hip joint and in the late stages there will be a flexion contracture of the hip, but early this is absent.

The diagnostic clue is the distortion of the psoas muscle on the AP x-ray film of the lumbar spine. A special KUB x-ray film with emphasis on the soft tissue density will make the muscle shadow difference on both sides much clearer.

Although the psoas abscess is an extremely rare entity, possi-

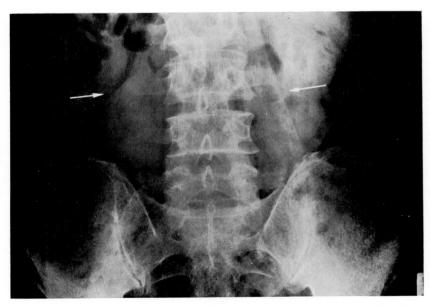

Figure 2B. Fever six weeks and vague left thigh pain. Psoas shadow markedly enlarged on one side as a result of a psoas abscess of hematogenous origin with no bony involvement, a difficult diagnosis to make. Only by viewing the films carefully will a diagnosis of psoas abscess be made.

bility of this type of infection must be remembered when there is vague pain in a thigh accompanied by spiking fever.

Meralgia Paresthetica

The person will complain of a vague type of pain that he has difficulty in specifying. He will say that the outside of his thigh feels as if "there are worms crawling there." When he touches some areas of his thigh, he obtains a disagreeable sensation. The pain is not severe; it is more annoying and worrisome than anything else. The cause is irritation of the lateral femoral cutaneous nerve. This peripheral nerve, which goes to the skin on the anterior and lateral aspect of the mid-thigh, is sensory only. It can be irritated by excessive fat in the pelvic area or it can be irritated by wearing a tight belt or tight corset. If other causes for neuritis are excluded, such as diabetic neuritis, radicular syndrome from the lumbar spine, or even tumors of the lumbar spine, the diagnosis of meralgia paresthetica should be entertained. The diagnosis is aided by injecting the anterior lip of the ilium with about 5 cc of 1% Xylocaine.® The disagreeable sensation on the thigh will commonly disappear. If one is convinced of the diagnosis, the injection should be repeated at intervals because the nerve has a variable course and only in this way can one be sure of having infiltrated the nerve.

Trochanteric Bursitis

Pain in the hip and leg area can be caused by bursitis of the greater torchanter. This affection is another of those that are overlooked not uncommonly. The patient complains of pain, often severe and acute, in the upper thigh and leg area. The pain may radiate all the way down to the knee. If the bursitis is of the acute variety, excruciating pain may be present that will prevent sleep. If the pain is of the more subacute or chronic type, it will of course be far less severe.

The examination will disclose tenderness, point, somewhere in the region of the greater trochanter. This tenderness is not necessarily over the greater trochanter but may be several inches away from it. The bursa extends for several inches distal and some for a few inches proximal to the greater trochanter, and any portion of the bursa may be the site of the inflammatory process.

If the bursitis is accompanied by calcification, it is more apt to be of the acute and very painful form rather than the more indolent subacute form.

There will be a complete range of motion of the hip joint but there may be slight pain at the extremes of internal rotation and of adduction. Of course, examination of the spine and the leg must be performed to exclude other causes of leg pain such asdisc syndrome, claudication from peripheral vascular disease, tumors, fractures, and so forth.

The x-ray films may or may not reveal a small area of soft tissue calcification near the greater torchanter.

The diagnosis is aided by injecting the tender area with a mixture of Xylocaine and corticosteroid and obtaining relief from the pain within twenty-four hours by this measure.

"Pigeon Toe" Gait in a Child
Intoeing gait, or "pigeon toes," is sometimes a confusing complaint. The intoeing gait of the small child is often caused not by adduction of the forefoot (pigeon toes) but by internal tibial torsion or femoral torsion. To differentiate the adducted forefoot from the internal rotation deformity of the tibia or femur, it is only necessary to examine the child's legs with him lying down. The normal foot will be seen to be well aligned in a straight position. In the child with internal tibial torsion, the axis of the ankle joint will be internally rotated in relation to the axis of the knee joint. If the child has femoral torsion or anteversion, there will be limitation of external rotation of the hip joint whereas internal rotation will be quite free and even possibly greater than normal. Furthermore, if femoral torsion or anteversion is present the greater torchanter of the femur will be felt more posterior than normal.

Congenital Dislocation of the Hip
Congenital dislocation of the hip is often overlooked. It can be overlooked even by the orthopedist if the child who is brought in for any problem other than for trauma is not examined for the possibility of a dislocated hip. In other words, every baby that is being examined for foot or any other complaint other than a

fracture should have his hips examined. It is sometimes not possible to examine the hips of a baby if the baby is screaming because of a fracture of the forearm, for instance, so that it is then
excusable to forego the hip examination for congenital dislocation of the hip until a later date. It goes without saying, however,
that every injured baby should have his hips examined to make
sure there is no fracture there also.

As a matter of fact, every newborn infant should have his hips
examined by his pediatrician to make sure that the hips are not
dislocated at birth. It is not possible to rely on x-ray films of the
hips; thus the clinical examination is of the utmost importance.
In the newborn baby, if the hip is dislocated there is contraction
of the adductor muscles on that side, so that the hip cannot be
abducted as far as the other side. Of course if both hips are
dislocated there is limitation of abduction on both sides, right
and left. The physician will find the presence of piston mobility
as he pulls the hip up and down towards the floor and towards
the ceiling if the hip is dislocated. When the physician abducts
the hip, the "click of Ortolani" is felt as the femur jumps in and
out of the shallow acetabulum. If these signs are felt and there
is still doubt as to the diagnosis, treatment must be started on the
presumptive diagnosis rather than for treatment to be delayed
until much later when the x-ray films will disclose the dislocation.

Avulsion of the Medial Collateral Ligament of the Knee

Avulsion of the medial collateral ligament is usually not difficult to diagnose. However, this injury is missed when it is accompanied by the more evident and dramatic fracture of the
lateral condyle of the tibia. Mason Hohl has pointed out the
frequency with which the internal lateral ligament of the knee
is ruptured when the lateral condyle of the tibia is fractured. If
this ligamentous injury is not diagnosed and repaired early, disabling instability of the knee will occur despite accurate reduction
of the tibial fracture. The diagnosis can be made by a stress AP
x-ray film taken of the knee with pressure made to distract the
medial side of the knee.

Undisplaced Fracture of the Proximal Tibia in Children

Fracture of the proximal end of the tibia in children can be misleading. Fracture here, even if it is undisplaced and incomplete, can lead to serious valgus deformity because of the stimulation to growth of the tibia when the fracture is close to the epiphyseal plate. The physician diagnoses this fracture as an innocuous one and promises the parents that the quickly healing tibia will result in no deformity. When the cast is removed, however, valgus deformity of moderate or severe degree can be present. It is important therefore to be aware of this possibility and at least to warn the parents of the possibility of deformity. In addition, slight overcorrection of the fracture with slight varus may be helpful if the potential valgus deformity is recognized.

Fractures of the Epiphyseal Plate of the Distal Femur or Proximal Tibia

Fractures through the epiphyseal plate of the distal femur or proximal tibia can be present and missed. The fracture can reduce itself, and of course the x-ray films will then be perfectly normal in both the AP and lateral views. It is only by being aware of the possibility of the fracture after an injury to the region and by taking a stress film with the knee abducted that the fracture line through the cartilaginous epiphyseal plate will be seen. Thus the leg will be immobilized and protected, and displacement of the fracture will be avoided.

Transient Synovitis of the Hip in Children

Transient synovitis of the hip is a well-known entity in children. It is difficult to distinguish this condition from early Legg-Perthes disease. The onset, and the clinical picture of the two conditions, is the same. Transient synovitis, however, usually occurs in smaller children under the age of three, whereas Legg-Perthes disease occurs in the later age group, usually from three to ten. One cannot, however, rely on the difference in age to make the diagnosis. The parents will say that the child has been limping for a few days. The child seems well systemically but the examiner will find some limitation of motion of the involved hip, especially in rotation and in abduction. Flexion is usually normal. X-ray films of the hip will disclose no abnormality. The blood count and sedimentation rate are usually normal also. It is only by observing the child over a period of one or several weeks that the condition can be distinguished from Legg-Perthes disease in the very early stages. True, Legg-Perthes disease even at the first x-ray film frequently discloses the usual flattening or change in density of the femoral head, but this is not invariably true. Naturally, suppurative arthritis of the hip must be distinguished from transient synovitis, but this usually is not difficult since in suppurative arthritis there is fever, leukocytosis, and much more pain. Aspiration of the hip joint will reveal the presence of pus in the hip if suppurative arthritis is present.

Recurrent Dislocation of the Patella
Recurrent dislocation of the patella is difficult to diagnose at

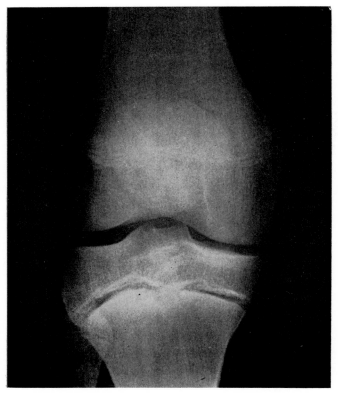

Figure 3A.   Pain in the knee after a motorcycle accident in a 14-year-old boy.

times. There is a history of a knee twist or injury of some sort, usually in a young person but at times in an adult. When the examiner sees the patient's knee, all he can find is a swollen, tender knee. There are several telltale findings, however, that will give one clues to the correct diagnosis. First, if the history is obtained in detail one finds a history of the kneecap going out to the side. There may in addition have been similar episodes in the past. Usually the patella reduces itself spontaneously, but at times the patient will say that he pushed the knee cap back into place.

When the knee is examined, one should test every such patient by having the patient sit on the examining table with his knees

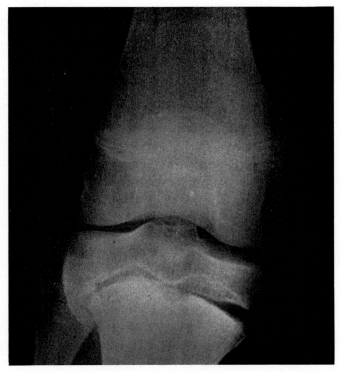

Figure 3B. Only by a stress film of the tibia is the displaced epiphysis seen. It is important to suspect epiphyseal subluxations in children who are injured.

flexed over the edge of the table. Then the examiner pushes the patella laterally. If the patella is unstable, this instability will be found by the patella being able to be moved laterally excessively. One should test the other knee for comparison, but it must be remembered that both knees may be unstable as far as the patella is concerned.

X-ray films can also give a clue. There may be a small flake fracture fragment seen in the knee joint. If a defect of the underside of the patella is seen in the lateral or tangential view of the patella, the diagnosis of recurrent dislocation of the patella is made stronger.

Charcot Joint

A Charcot knee joint in its earliest stages can be mistaken for a torn medial meniscus or other derangement. The patient with a Charcot knee has a history which is similar to that of the patient with an injured meniscus. He states that his knee is unstable, that it locks, that it gives way, and that it swells. Although it is commonly assumed that the patient with a Charcot knee has no pain, this is not always the case. There may be pain in the patient with a neuropathic knee joint. In the early stages, x-ray films may be normal or there may be very little disorganization of the knee joint found on the x-ray film. The correct diagnosis may be made by eliciting a history of stiffness, by absence of patellar and Achilles reflexes, and by the absence of normal pupillary reflexes of the eye. Because diabetes can cause neuropathic joints, a query for diabetes must be made. Diagnosis can be verified by obtaining spinal fluid with serologic examination of it and by having a glucose tolerance test made for diabetes.

Syningomyelia and congenital insensitivity to pain are two other disorders that can cause neuropathic joints.

Suppurative Arthritis

In the infant, this condition of pus in the hip joint is overlooked not uncommonly. The infection can be derived from an infected ear, from infections of the respiratory tract, or from the urinary tract. It is days and usually weeks before the diagnosis is made. The infant will be irritable and there is usually high fever, but in some instances the fever is not very great.

It is only by examining the motion of the hip joint and noticing that the infant resents having his leg moved, that one suspects the diagnosis of a septic hip. On further examination, one finds tenderness and swelling in the region of the hip. The white blood cell count and sedimentation rate are found to be elevated. X-ray films usually are normal until late in the disease when there is evidence of destruction of the joint and bone. The diagnosis is ascertained by aspirating the hip joint and obtaining pus.

In the elderly, suppurative arthritis of any joint can be present and there is often deceptively little in the way of systemic symptoms. Fever may be nonexistent and the white blood cell count may not be elevated significantly. It is not known why elderly people are more prone to develop hematogenous septic joints than are young people. It is extremely important to make the diagnosis of septic joint in these elderly people because if the mistaken diagnosis of synovitis or degenerative arthritis is made, cortisone may be injected and this will make the infection worse, of course.

It need hardly be mentioned that in infants and children suppurative arthritis may occur in any joint of the body, and in the small infant the diagnosis will be made only by scrutinizing both arms and both legs and the rest of the body, carefully looking for swelling, limitation of motion of a joint, increased heat, as well as systemic signs of infection.

Resistant Rickets

Resistant rickets is another clinical entity of importance because it is mistaken for congenital deformities of the legs, such as dyschondroplasia. If the diagnosis of resistant rickets is missed, the opportunity to treat the condition medically with high doses of Vitamin D is lost. Furthermore, unnecessary surgery can be performed and recurrence of the deformity after a surgery will invariably take place if the patient is not diagnosed correctly and is not given Vitamin D.

When the child is seen, there is usually some deformity of the legs, either varus or valgus. The x-ray picture of rickets, including widening of the epiphyseal cartilaginous plate and metaphyseal irregularity, is present to a variable degree.

The diagnosis is substantiated by finding abnormalities of the blood chemically, especially alkaline phosphatase, which is markedly elevated. The serum calcium is usually normal or slightly lower than normal, and the serum phosphorus is usually lower than normal. The diagnosis is also aided by seeing the response both clinically and radiologically with massive doses of Vitamin D.

Reiter's Syndrome

Reiter's syndrome is frequently misdiagnosed. Because the onset is acute and the patient complains of a very painful, swollen, hot joint, one usually suspects suppurative arthritis, gonorrheal arthritis, osteomyelitis, or early rheumatoid arthritis.

Most frequently affected are the knees, ankles, and feet. Several joints may be affected.

The x-ray films often reveal some characteristic periosteal changes near the joint. The calcaneus shows, typically, some erosions and some plantar calcaneal spurs.

Diagnosis is aided by eliciting a history of urethritis and conjunctivitis. The latter components of the disease often precede the arthritis by several weeks or months.

Fibrosis of the Vastus Intermedius

Fibrosis of the vastus intermedius is seen in children as a cause of limitation of flexion of the knees. The child will be brought in by the mother because he has a stiff knee which he has not been able to flex ever since he was an infant. The mother and often the doctor will think that this is a congenital affection. It is in fact caused by the child having received intramuscular injections when he was an infant, the injections having been given into the thigh muscles, resulting in contracture of the extensor muscles of the knee. If the diagnosis is made correctly, surgical treatment consisting of excision of the vastus intermedius muscle and fibrous tissue will often result in improvement in the range of flexion of the knee.

Bipartite Patella

The bipartite patella is another condition that is easily confused. It is often misdiagnosed as a fracture. The radiologic appearance of the bipartite patella is diagnostic, however, and the diagnosis can be made even if there is tenderness and some swelling over the patella when the knee has been injured. The bipartite fragment is of course congenital and it is not a fracture. It is always in the outer upper quadrant of the patella. The edges of the partition are quite regular and smooth, in contradistinction to a fracture. Once in a while there is a tripartite patella where more than one fragment is present in addition to the main body of the patella. In such a case the fragments are in the upper outer quadrant of the patella and the edges again are smooth.

THE BACK

Carcinoma of the Pancreas

One uncommon cause of back pain that is probably missed more frequently than not is *carcinoma of the pancreas*. The pain of carcinoma of the pancreas is often in the back, so that the orthopedic surgeon may be the first physician who sees the patient. It is only when the patient becomes jaundiced that the diagnosis of carcinoma of the head of the pancreas is made. Because the disease occurs in elderly patients in whom there is some degenerative arthritis of the spine, the diagnosis of carcinoma of the pancreas is confused with the nonsymptomatic arthritic condition. In the patients with carcinoma of the pancreas, there is no pain accompanying motion of the spine even though there may be some limitation of motion as a result of the degenerative changes that are present there. There is no tenderness on percussion of the spine. When the patient lies down in bed, there is little if any relief of pain. Even though the internist will report that the barium enema and GI series are reported to be normal, one should ask for other studies such as enzyme studies and liver studies to make sure that pancreatic carcinoma does not exist.

Primary Tumors of the Spine

It is well known that primary tumors of the spine and its environs may cause back pain. Many patients are seen who have back pain resulting from a primary tumor of the spine whose diagnosis is missed for a long time. Such laboratory investigation as sedimentation rate and uric acid examination are minimum requirements for any patient who complains of back pain of more than a few days' duration. Of course if a history or physical examination so indicates any other laboratory tests such as albumin, globulin, and serum electrophoresis, examination of the urine and a complete blood count may be necessary.

In any event, if persistent pain is present and despite the

absence of any abnormal neurological findings on the examination, a spinal puncture with or without a myelogram should be performed.

Metastatic Carcinoma

Metastatic carcinoma to the spine is a common cause of continued pain in the back. Because of the increased number of elderly patients now alive, this diagnosis is to be considered commonly. One of the most important aids in determining the presence of metastatic carcinoma to the spine is the history. The patient who has pain that has been present longer than a few days must be questioned regarding his or her past history. Some patients are ashamed of having had cancer and even to their physician they are reluctant to disclose such a history. The doctor must prod the patient into disclosing a history of cancer. If the patient has ever had cancer of any type in his history, he or she should be suspected of having a metastasis until absolute proof is present that none is there. In the diagnosis of metastatic malignancy the presence of bone tenderness, over a small area of bone, is helpful, and again the presence of pain at rest and at night is important. These people have more pain at rest than they do when they are up, although there is some pain when they move. Motion of the spine may not be restricted. The x-ray examination of the spine is of great significance. The x-ray films must be of good quality, and they should include the dorsal and the lumbar spine as well as the pelvis if there is any pain in the lower back area. Films often should be viewed in a bright light to see if some of the bones that are not dense, such as a transverse process or one of the lower ribs or the spinous process, show any osteolytic areas. If the pain persists, x-ray films should be made again within a matter of one, two, or three weeks and the films should be repeated again.

The laboratory findings can be very significant, and increased alkaline phosphatase, an increase in the blood calcium, and an increased sedimentation rate could be significant. If these people when questioned will relate in their history that they do not feel well generally, that their appetite has diminished and there may be a recent loss of weight, metastatic carcinoma may be present.

Cervical Disc Syndrome

One cause of lower back pain that is uncommon is a cervical disc syndrome without any neck or arm symptoms. There can be pressure on the spinal cord in the cervical spine by arthritic or degenerative disc changes. This pressure may be exerted in such a manner that pain in the lower back and legs only will be felt. This condition admittedly is quite rate, inasmuch as cervical syndromes will almost invariably cause pain in the neck and arms. It is therefore important in obscure low back and leg pain of continued duration to obtain films of the cervical spine and a cervical myelogram in addition to other data that is obtained.

Parkinson's Disease

Parkinson's disease (paralysis agitans) is a cause of low back pain that is overlooked by some physicians. Back pain, as a matter of fact, may be the first symptom that brings the patient with early Parkinson's disease to the orthopedic surgeon. The cause of pain in Parkinson's disease is the rigidity of the musculature of the back causing stiffness in the small joints of the lumbar and dorsal spine, and these become partially rigid after a few weeks and months. Therefore the patient experiences pain as a result of the enforced limitation of motion of the small joints of the spine as well as because of the stretching of the contracted and tightened musculature. The pain is augmented by degenerative changes in the spine which often are present in the same age group where Parkinson's disease occurs. Diagnosis is made by the lack of normal facial expression change, by the intention tremor or rigidity of the arms or legs, and by the limitation of motion and rigid manner of movement of the lumbar spine. In such a patient, confirmation is obtained through a thorough neurological examination.

Intermittent Claudication of the Spinal Cord

Intermittent claudication of the spinal cord, or cauda equina, is another syndrome causing somewhat obscure pain in the back and legs. These patients complain of pain in their back or upper thighs and back when they walk. The pain is relieved on standing or resting. This type of pain is very similar to the intermittent claudication that is seen in claudication of the legs.

There are two mechanisms by which claudication of the cord takes place. In one, there is ischemia by inadequate arterial supply of the cord or cauda equina. This becomes symptomatic as the patient walks and the blood supply to the cord or cauda becomes lessened by the increased flow of blood to the legs. The other mechanism is by increased edema of the nerve roots from irritation as the patient is active when walking. Sometimes it is very difficult to distinguish between these two causes of claudication.

Backache in Children

When a child complains of back pain and scoliosis or lateral curvature is present, one should suspect a tumor, either benign or malignant. The most common benign tumor that causes pain in the spine with scoliosis is osteoid osteoma. This small benign tumor can be present in any portion of the spine, or in any bone for that matter. The small area of sclerosis or a central area of diminished density is often remote from the area of pain so that one must search for it by taking x-ray films of the entire spine and pelvis. Typically, the child or adolescent will state that he is relieved of his pain with aspirin. The pain is often worse at night.

Other tumors, malignant or benign, may occur in children, such as lymphomas or aneursymal bone cysts. In small children, probably the most common tumor of the spine causing pain would be a *Wilm's tumor* or *neuroblastoma*. Examination of the child's abdomen may elicit the presence of a mass there. X-ray films, of course, must be taken to see if a destructive lesion of the spine is present. Osteomyelitis of the spine is not common but it occurs in children especially and can cause pain there. The diagnosis of osteomyelitis of the spine is usually not too difficult. If there is fever and the onset is acute, early x-ray films do not disclose any abnormality, but repeated x-ray films at intervals will show the sclerosis that accompanies osteomyelitis in the bones of the spine. The other signs of infection, of course, are usuallly present. These include an elevated sedimentation rate, leukocytosis, and so forth. In some instances, especially in adults, systemic signs of infection such as fever and elevated sedimentation rate may be minimal. The more unusual types of chronic infection, such as undulant fever, typhoid, and paratyphoid fever, are not particularly prone to attack the spine in children, but they can do so. Where the progress of the disease is slower, then one must consider such conditions as coccidioidomycosis and the other chronic infections, including, of course, tuberculosis. Tests for these diseases, such as the tuberculin test, the coccidioidomycosis skin test, and agglutination tests of the blood, will reveal significant data in the presence of these chronic infections.

INDOLENT INFECTION OF THE DISC SPACE. Discitis occurs in children for some reason much more frequently than it does in adults. These indolent infections are difficult to diagnose inasmuch as there is no fever and very little of the very few other signs associated with infection. There may be some elevation of the sedimentation rate and this may be the only generalized reaction to the infection.

RUPTURED INTERVERTEBRAL DISC. This occurs in children much more often than is generally known. The child of nine or ten who complains of pain in his leg is often thought to have what is called "growing pains," whereas on close examination the patient can be found to have a ruptured intervertebral disc. The pain can continue and if there are abnormal neurological findings such as diminished Achilles or patellar reflexes with some toe weakness and hypesthesia one should be alert enough to order a myelogram which will show the abnormality or defect in the spinal canal. Incidentally, the children who are operated upon for ruptured intervertebral discs do better as a general rule than adults because there are fewer neuroses in children. Finally, in this vein, it is possible that children who have what has been termed disc space infection of a chronic nature, or "discitis," may really be suffering from a form of ruptured intervertebral disc of a central type.

DISLOCATION OF THE APOPHYSIS OR EPIPHYSIS OF THE VERTEBRAL BODY. These youngsters will reveal a history of very arduous weight lifting, and the epiphyseal plates of one or several of the vertebrae can separate from the vertebral body as a result of this tremendous force. The teenage boy will complain of progressive weakness and numbness of his leg and he will say that his back is painful as well. The x-ray film may disclose one or several of the epiphyseal plates to be slightly displaced from the remainder of the vertebral body. A myelogram will provide evidence of impingement of the epiphysis within the spinal canal pressing on the spinal cord or cauda equina. Incidentally, such youngsters respond well to laminectomy.

Pain in the Upper Back

Pain in the upper back is commonly misdiagnosed. The most common cause of pain in the upper back is a *cervical disc syndrome,* inasmuch as the pain from the cervical spine is referred to the upper dorsal spine as well as into the arm. Examination of the cervical spine will reveal in such instances limitation of motion, especially in extension, and there will be pain accompanying the motion, the pain being referred to the upper back area. Naturally, other causes for pain in the upper spine must be eliminated. These include tumors, fractures, especially pathologic fractures, and also infections.

WINGED SCAPULA. This is another cause for pain in the upper back. A winged scapula is caused by weakness of the serratus magnus muscle which in turn is the result of a traction injury of the long thoracic nerve of Bell. This nerve may be injured by carrying a heavy weight on the shoulder or by lifting something very heavy, thus stretching this rather vulnerable nerve. There is tenderness in such instances along the vertebral border of the scapula, and the scapula will be seen to wing as the arm is abducted.

BRAIN TUMOR. Pain in the neck and upper back region can also be caused by a brain tumor, and where no local causes for pain in the neck and upper back area are found, a thorough neurological examination must be made and repeated at intervals to make sure that a brain tumor is not present. In such instances there will be a normal range of cervical and spinal motion, there will be no local tenderness, and x-ray films of the cervical and dorsal spine will, of course, be normal.

Low Back Pain

The patient who has low back pain often presents a difficult problem for diagnosis. If he has been operated upon and a laminectomy has been performed, a myelogram should be done on the patient's spine since the possibility exists that pain from a *postoperative meningocele* may be causative. The surgeon at the time of the spine operation may not be aware that the dura has been punctured. Postoperatively, a sack of tissue surrounding the spinal fluid can be the cause of vague but continued pain in the back or leg.

If a patient with low back pain complains of back and leg pain for many months, and even if there is reason to suspect him to be *hysterical, neurotic,* or even *malingering,* a myelogram is indicated because ruptured discs or benign tumors may be present, with neurotic syndromes superimposed on the organic disease. In this vein, it should be remembered that coccydynia, pain in the coccyx, of chronic nature, usually considered to be neurotic, is often caused by a ruptured intervertebral disc with nerve root irritation.

In males of middle age or older, a rectal examination may reveal the cause of pain to be *carcinoma of the prostate* which would indicate the possibility that metastasis to the spine is the most probable cause of the patient's pain.

An x-ray film of the pelvis may reveal the cause of vague back pain to be rheumatoid spondylitis by seeing irregularity of the sacroiliac joints.

Physiological Dislocation of the Cervical Spine in Children

Dislocation of the second or the third cervical vertebra in children is a diagnosis that is erroneously made. The spine at this region is normally hypermobile in children, and some degree of subluxation is therefore normal. A child with the x-ray films showing this displacement should not be harassed by hospitalization, traction, etc. The diagnosis of physiologic displacement of the second or the third cervical vertebra is made when there is no history of severe trauma and when the clinical picture reveals only slight limitation of motion of this portion of the spine, usually because of soft tissue injury or infection.

Morquio's Disease and Hurler's Disease

Morquio's disease is very easily confused with Hurler's disease. These are both diseases of mucopolysaccharide series of carbohydrate abnormality involving the cartilage and other mesothelial structures.

It is important to differentiate the two diseases inasmuch as the Morquio patients have a far better prognosis than do the Hurler cases. When an infant is seen, therefore, one must know which of the two is present because of the far worse prognosis for longevity of Hurler's disease and because of the diminished mentality of the Hurler patient.

Possibly the easiest method of differentiating the two diseases is by the appearance of the spine on the x-ray films. A lateral

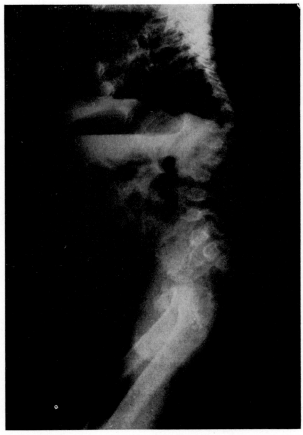

Figure 4A.   Hurler's disease in a 4-year-old female. Kyphosis at the dorsal-lumbar junction is present and there is inferior beaking of the vertebrae at the site of kyphosis. It is of some importance to differentiate Hurler's from Morquio's disease.

view of the spine in Morquio's disease will show multiple flattened vertebrae with central beaking of the vertebra plana type. In Hurler's disease there is inferior beaking with ovoid bodies seen on the lateral views.

There are many other distinguishing features, including the fact that in Hurler's disease there is excretion of chondrotin sulfate and heparitin sulfate in the urine, characteristic large bulging head, flat nose, flared nostrils, short neck, kyphosis, and corneal

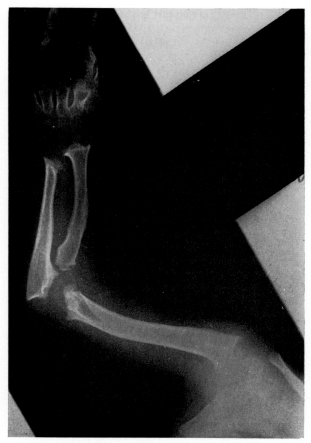

Figure 4B. Hurler's disease, forearm of the same child. The diaphysis of the radius and ulna are thickened and there is tapering of the distal ulna as well as shortening and proximal tapering of the metacarpals. Osteoporosis of the distal metacarpal bones is seen.

opacity. There are in addition glanulations in the leukocytes in many patients.

Other varieties of the two diseases, called the San Fillipo, Sheie, Maroteaux, Lamy disease are of more academic importance.

Cervical Cord Contusion

In older patients who are involved in automobile accidents, contusion of the cervical spinal cord is a condition that is not uncommonly overlooked. These people have stiff cervical spines so that when they are involved in an automobile accident the jarring

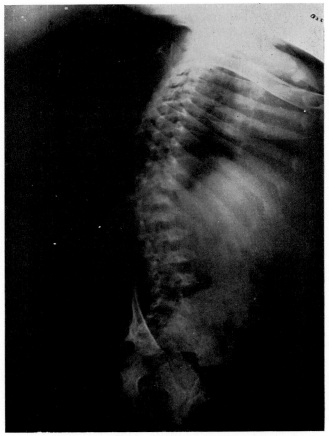

Figure 5A. Morquio's disease. Dorsal-lumbar kyphosis is present. The vertebrae demonstrate central beaking contrasted with the inferior beaking of the vertebral bodies of Hurler's disease.

that they get from the impact stretches the cervical portion of the spinal cord. Their cervical spine is stiff, and without any fracture or dislocation this excessive stretching of the spinal cord encased in an almost rigid cervical spine is enough to cause extensive neurological abnormalities.

When the x-ray films are taken and no overt evidence of trauma is seen, in other words when there is no evidence of dislocation or fracture, the examiner may think the patient is malingering when he complains of tingling, numbness, and weakness of his arm or leg. When a careful neurological examination is performed, however, there may be found signs of long tract cord damage. Babinski reflexes may be found, and there will be anatomically consistent patterns of hypesthesia and segmental weak-

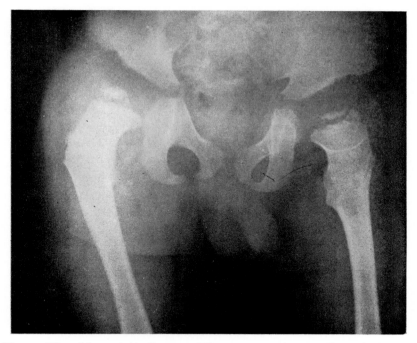

Figure 5B. Morquio's disease. The same patient. There is irregularity and flattening of the femoral capital epiphyses. Also irregularity of the ossification centers of the greater trochanter is present. The femoral necks are shortened and thickened and the acetabulae are irregular.

ness of muscle groups. If the signs are not too abnormal, the patient will recover with a period of rest for the cervical spine and the cervical spinal cord.

Another trap that the unwary physician may fall into is one of fracture or dislocation in the lower cervical and upper dorsal spine. This area is often missed on routine x-ray films, and significant injuries here can be present after trauma of various types. Therefore, it is important to order x-ray films in any suspected case of injury in this region or this hidden area by suitably positioned views (Swinner's position) of the cervical dorsal junction.

Patients with rheumatoid arthritis who are involved in even minor automobile accidents or who sustain falls can sustain a

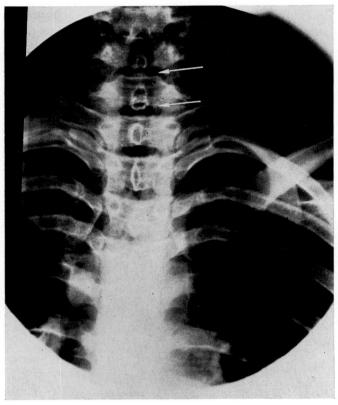

Figure 6A. Pain in neck after "whiplash." Careful examination of AP view shows spinous processes of C6 and C7 to be separated.

dislocation of the first and second vertebrae. As a matter of fact, dislocations between these two vertebrae, namely between the atlas and the axis, can occur without any trauma merely by the destructive process of rheumatoid disease. The rheumatoid arthritic patient who complains of pain in his neck should therefore have adequately clear x-ray films of the upper cervical spine to make sure there is no such dislocation present. If the subluxation or dislocation is not discovered, such a patient may suddenly impinge the proximal portion of the cervical cord and die instantly.

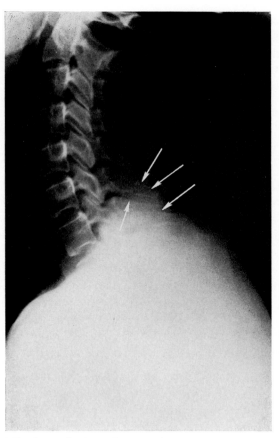

Figure 6B. The lateral view shows a fracture at the base of the spinous process of C6 in this film.

THE ARM

Pancoast Tumors

Pancoast tumors (superior pulmonary sulcus tumors) can masquerade as bursitis of the shoulder. The patient with such a tumor of the lung will complain of vague pain in the shoulder and arm. X-ray films of the shoulder may indeed show a calcified area adjacent to the greater tuberosity, and this is the area that is treated. The cause of the pain can, however, be a malignant tumor of the superior portion of the lung, and films of the lung should be made if the patient of middle age or older complains of pain in the arm that does not respond to local treatment.

Primary or Secondary Bone Tumors

Primary or secondary bone tumors can be mistaken for tendinitis or bursitis of the shoulder area. Adequate x-ray films of the bone in the region prevent making such a mistake.

Suppurative Arthritis or Suppurative Subdeltoid Bursitis

Suppurative arthritis or suppurative subdeltoid bursitis of the shoulder can mistakenly be treated for the common acute or chronic tendinitis or bursitis. The patient with acute hematogenous suppurative arthritis or bursitis will have severe pain. Usually ths entity occurs in older people for some reason, rather than in young people. If the shoulder area is swollen and is very tender and the patient complains of unusually severe pain, the anterior aspect of the shoulder should be aspirated to see if purulent material is obtained. In no case should injection of steroids be made when one suspects suppurative arthritis.

Supracondylar Fractures of the Humerus

Supracondylar fractures of the humerus are easily missed in small infants. The reason is that there is so little of the distal end of the humerus that is ossified that x-ray films are misleading. The x-ray films will show nothing abnormal except some soft tissue swelling, and there may be some slight malalignment of the forearm in relation to the humerus. This can be misinterpreted as a dislocation, and a perfunctory attempt at a reduction may erroneously be made. The elbow is usually immobilized with a splint or in a sling, but it is only months after the injury has taken place, when there is growth of the lower humerus and ossification becomes evident of the lower epiphysis of the humerus, that the true nature of the injury becomes apparent. I believe it is extremely rare for an elbow dislocation to occur in a small infant under the age of one year, and much more common is a fracture of the distal end of the humerus through the cartilaginous epiphysis.

Injuries to the Median, Radial, and Ulnar Nerves

Injuries to the median, radial, and ulnar nerves occur accompanying supracondylar fractures *in children* and these are not easy to detect. The child of three or four is not an easy person to examine for nerve injuries of the hand. The small child with an injury to the elbow is in pain, and it is only after a prolonged and patient attempt at a detailed examination of the motor function of the nerves to the hand that injuries to these nerves

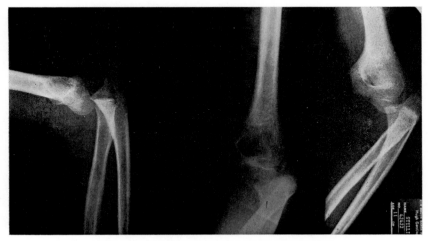

Figure 7A. Fracture of the medial epicondyle of the humerus with the fragment displaced into the joint. The elbow joint is dislocated. Intra-articularly displaced fractures of the medial epicondyle are frequently overlooked in such injuries.

will be found. I do not have to emphasize the importance of detecting the existence of an injured median nerve, for instance, so that proper treatment, even if it is only diminution of pressure around the median nerve, is instituted early.

Volkman's Contracture of the Forearm

Volkman's contracture of the forearm is also an entity that is usually missed in its early stages. Of course these injuries occur usually after fractures of the elbow region. What is not so well known is that, in addition to the possibility of this condition after

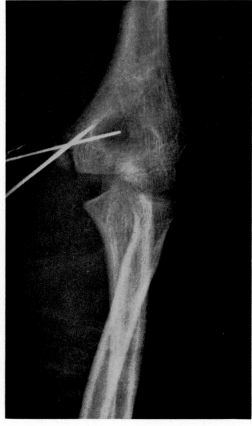

Figure 7B.   After open reduction and retrieval of the epicondyle with reduction of the dislocation of the elbow.

elbow injuries and injuries of the proximal forearm, it can occur after injuries to the wrist. Therefore, it is important to suspect all children who have severe injuries anywhere in the elbow, forearm, or wrist area of developing Volkman's contracture.

The earliest sign or symptom of Volkman's contracture is pain. This complication of injuries to the arm can be present despite a

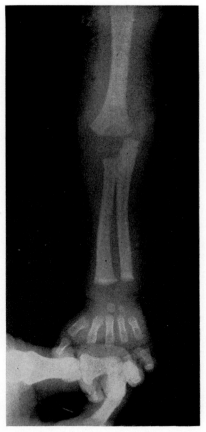

Figure 8A. AP view of the elbow of a 6-month-old baby who fell from his crib. It would seem there is medial dislocation of the elbow joint. When the elbow was opened, a fracture through the distal humeral epiphysis was found with complete displacement of the epiphysis. Elbow dislocations in babies are extremely rare. It is more common to have fractures through the cartilaginous epiphysis.

palpable radial pulse and despite normal sensation to the fingers. Many textbooks state that the first sign of Volkman's contracture is absence of the pulse and absence of sensation. This statement is not true. In addition to pain that is unusually severe for an injury to the forearm, in the presence of Volkman's contracture there is universally pain on attempts to extend the fingers either passively or actively. The diagnosis of this complication is, needless, to say, of the utmost importance at the earliest possible time for effective control.

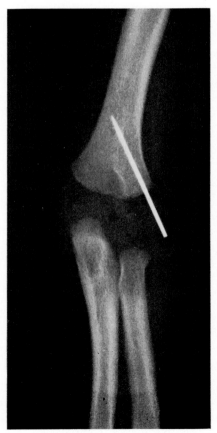

Figure 8B.   After open reduction and fixation of the epiphyseal fracture.

Anterior Interosseous Nerve Palsy

Anterior interosseous nerve palsy with weakness of some of the flexor muscles of the fingers is another entity that is easily missed. It is only by frequently testing the flexor muscles of the fingers that this entity can be diagnosed following injury of the forearm or elbow.

Olecranon Bursitis

Olecranon bursitis is an innocuous affair usually. It can, however, be the first sign of gout. Every person, I believe, who has swelling with accompanying pain in the region of the olecranon process should have a blood uric acid determination inasmuch as the ordinary type of swelling over the olecranon process, namely

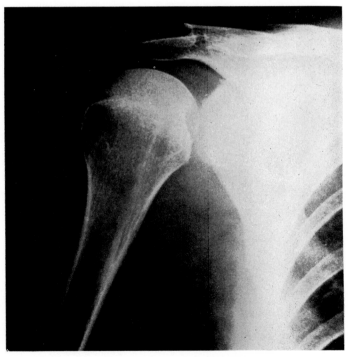

Figure 9A. Posterior dislocation of the shoulder joint. In the AP view, lack of normal overlap of the head of the humerus on the glenoid is a suspicious finding of posterior dislocation of the shoulder joint.

bursitis, is painless. Another thing to remember is that bursitis of the olecranon process can easily become suppurative, so that if there is any local evidence of inflammation, the physician must be wary of injecting corticostedoids into the bursa since this would make the infection worse.

Posterior Dislocation of the Shoulder

Posterior dislocation of the shoulder is a diagnostic trap. The more common anterior dislocation is easily diagnosed both clinically and by x-ray. The more uncommon posterior dislocation,

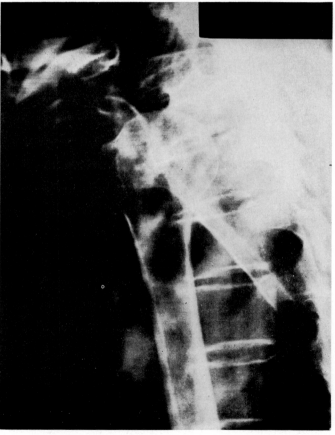

Figure 9B. The lateral transthoracic view of the shoulder reveals a posteriorly displaced head of the humerus in relation to the glenoid.

however, is often missed on the x-ray film. It is commonly present after injury to the shoulder as a result of a convulsion, either epileptic or from electric shock. The best method of making the diagnosis is by clinical examination, and then it can be verified by proper x-ray films. Every patient who has an injured shoulder should be examined while he is sitting. The physician should then look down upon the shoulder and at the same time feel the shoulder. He will both see and feel that the prominent humeral head is posteriorly displaced if there is a dislocation of the humeral head posteriorly. Then the properly taken x-ray films in the

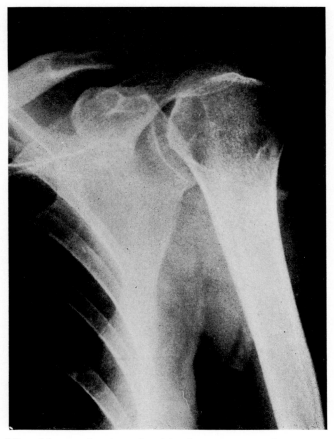

Figure 9C. After reduction the AP view now reveals a more normal overlap of the humeral head on the glenoid.

axillary and in the transthoracic positions will corroborate the diagnosis.

Subluxation of the Shoulder

Subluxation of the shoulder is a condition that occurs in young people after injury. The shoulder joint is painful and no abnormality can be detected on the x-ray film. The condition occurs after an initial severe injury to the shoulder whereby the anterior capsule is torn. The young person who complains of pain in the shoulder following a fall on his arm will have very few abnormal

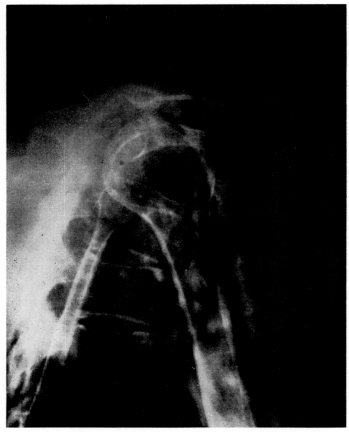

Figure 9D. After reduction the lateral transthoracic view now reveals the normal relationship of the head of the humerus to the glenoid.

findings on examination of the region. One finding, however, is universally present. Pain is present on passive attempts to rotate the shoulder externally. The patient must be examined thoroughly to make sure that no other injury is present. If all entities, such as rupture of the supraspinatus, the biceps, and articular fractures, are ruled out and if the pain persists for a number of weeks, the diagnosis of recurrent subluxation of the shoulder is made. This is not the same thing as recurrent *dislocation*. The only treatment for this condition is surgical, so that the diagnosis is important.

Congenital Recurrent Dislocation of the Shoulder

Congenital recurrent dislocation of the shoulder is another shoulder affection that is easily missed. It can easily be mistaken for the usual simple post-traumatic recurrent dislocation. Con-

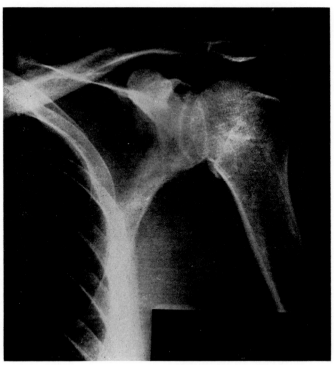

Figure 10A. A 67-year-old man fell after having a convulsion. AP view of the shoulder reveals no gross abnormality.

genital recurrent dislocation is the result of a congenitally loose capsule of the joint. It takes little or no trauma to dislocate the shoulder, and in fact the patient if he is asked to can dislocate his shoulder at will. This condition is very difficult to treat and should not be operated, since it is only a matter of neurotic concern for the patient. It is not disabling as is the more common acquired recurrent dislocation of the shoulder.

Dislocations of the Semilunar Bone of the Wrist

Dislocations of the semilunar bone of the wrist are not always

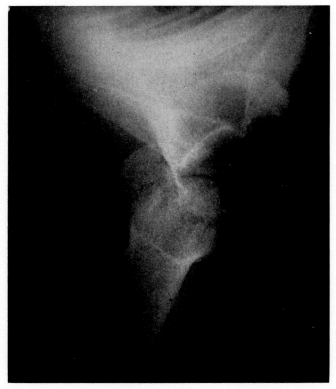

Figure 10B.   Axillary view of the shoulder taken at the same time reveals posterior dislocation of the humeral head. This emphasizes the importance of taking films in the axillary position as well as the transthoracic position in patients in whom posterior dislocation is suspected by clinical examination.

easy to discern. After a wrist injury, diagnosis of sprain is often made where a dislocation of one of the carpal bones exists, most commonly the semilunar. In some emergency hospitals, x-ray films that are made after an injury are not the best. A physician should insist on a straight lateral view of the wrist as well as a straight AP view and an oblique view. If there is any doubt about the existence of a dislocation or subluxation, comparable views of the opposite normal wrist must be made. In the AP view of

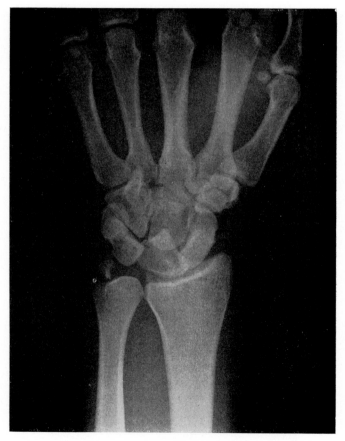

Figure 11A. AP view of a 19-year-old man who injured his wrist after a motorcycle accident. A triangular appearance of the semilunar bone should make one suspicious of a dislocation of that bone. The fracture of the ulnar styloid process is incidental.

the wrist, the dislocated semilunar bone has the appearance of a triangle replacing the normal rectangular appearance of the bone. This is a good clue to the fact that the bone is dislocated, and a lateral view will show the dislocation more clearly.

Thoracic Outlet Syndromes

Thoracic outlet syndromes are not common but can be mistaken for radicular syndromes of the cervical spine. The Adson sign, namely obliteration of the radial pulse on rotation of the cervical spine in deep inspiration, diminution of the radial pulse

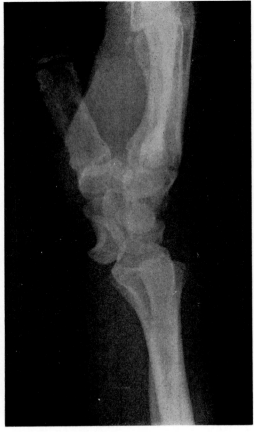

Figure 11B.   The straight lateral view of the wrist confirms the diagnosis of dislocation of the semilunar bone.

on hyperabduction or on retraction of the shoulders, will help in making the diagnosis of a thoracic outlet syndrome. Of course the presence of a cervical rib on the x-ray films plus the presence of the signs clinically of thoracic outlet syndrome mentioned above will help in making the diagnosis. Finally, the vascular surgeon may perform an arteriogram to confirm the diagnosis of this syndrome.

Carpal Tunnel Syndrome

Carpal tunnel syndrome is a common cause of complaint of pain, numbness, and tingling in the hand. The usual story of onset of these symptoms in middle-aged women is well known. The pain comes on at night when the wrists are relaxed, and the

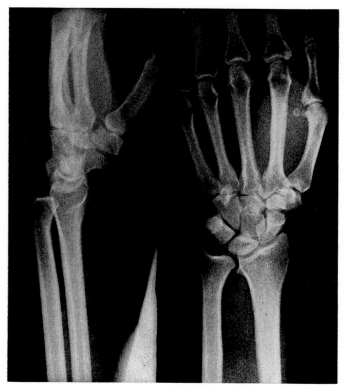

Figure 12A. Routine views of the wrist in a 31-year-old woman who fell on her hand. No fracture is seen.

volar carpal ligament then presses upon the median nerve more. On examination, of course, there is diminished sensation over the thumb, index and middle fingers. In the later cases there is even atrophy and weakness of the thenar muscles. Other possible causes for dysesthesia of the hand are eliminated by further examination. These other causes of dysesthesia of the hand are cervical disc syndromes, radicular pains from lesions and diseases of the upper arm, and even tumors in the chest cage such as Pancoast. The

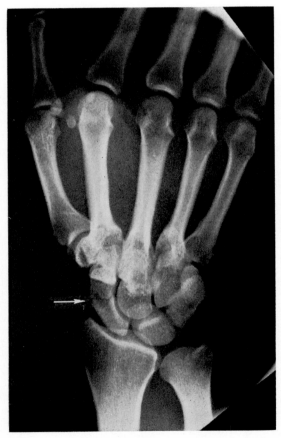

Figure 12B. AP view with the hand in ulnar deviation reveals the presence of a transverse fracture of the navicular bone. Such a view should be taken in addition to the routine ones in suspected fractures of the navicular.

examiner may be led astray from making the correct diagnosis of carpal tunnel syndrome by the presence of pain in the forearm or even in the upper arm and shoulder accompanying the tingling and pain in the hand. In carpal tunnel syndrome there can be pain referred all the way from the fingers to the shoulder area. Cervical disc syndromes, epicondylitis of the elbow, and carpal tunnel syndromes often coexist so that the diagnosis becomes quite complicated, but it is necessary to find which of the syndromes is responsible for most of the symptoms.

Cervical Disc Syndromes

Cervical disc syndromes are quite commonly the cause of pain in the upper extremity. The pain in these syndromes can be very severe, and the important thing to remember is that x-ray films of the cervical spine can be quite normal. There may be severe and prolonged pain, and yet when one takes x-ray films one may

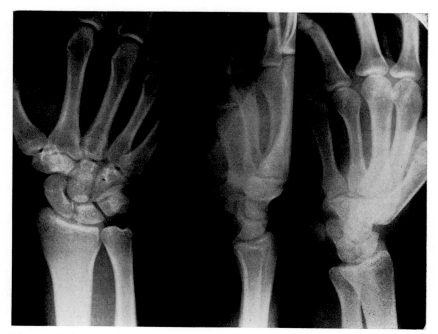

Figure 13A. Persistent pain in a hand for many months after a fall on an outstretched hand.

be mistaken as far as the diagnosis is concerned in that there may be no evidence of any arthritic spurring or other changes of the disc spaces on the films. Abnormal neurological findings, such as absence of triceps or biceps reflexes, may be present with weakness of the small muscles of the hand despite normal x-ray films. It is not too uncommon also to have other semi-acute or chronic affections accompanying cervical disc syndromes. These are calcified tendinitis of the shoulder, epicondylitis of the elbow, and carpal tunnel syndromes. It becomes confusing when two or three of these syndromes are present in the same patient, but one must then distinguish which is the major factor as the cause of the symptoms. Furthermore, at times it becomes necessary when one realizes there is more than one cause of the pain to treat several of them at the same time.

Winged Scapula
Winged scapula as a cause of vague pain in the shoulder is another entity that is missed frequently. This has been described elsewhere, but it is worth emphasizing here in a section on chronic pain in the arm. One should look for the abnormal prominence of the scapula posteriorly on elevation of the arm to distinguish this syndrome from others causing pain in the shoulder region.

Aneurysms of the Radial or Ulnar Arteries
Aneurysms of the radial or ulnar arteries in the palm of the hand are not common, but when they appear their diagnosis is

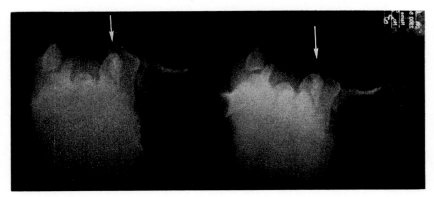

Figure 13B. Only by taking carpal tunnel view as shown in the two films above is the fracture of the greater multangular bone seen.

usually missed. There is vague pain in the hand, in the palm, and there is tenderness here. The patient is usually thought to be neurotic. There may or may not be a history of trauma before the onset of pain. If one palpates gently and carefully, one will feel an arterial thrill, and when one auscultates one will hear a bruit. If these findings are present, it then becomes easy to make the diagnosis by having an arteriogram made.

Sprain of the First Carpal-Metacarpal Joint

Sprain of the first carpal-metacarpal joint is another condition that is frequently missed. This condition occurs mainly in women and it is very easily confused with tenovaginitis of the abductor and extensor tendons at the radial styloid process, namely de Quervain's disease. In sprain of the first carpal-metacarpal joint, tenderness is directly over this joint instead of over the radial styloid process as in the tendinitis of de Quervain's disease. When the examiner attempts to move the first carpal-metacarpal passively, he elicits pain by so doing. Finkelstein's sign for de Quervain's disease is negative. This sign is elicted by asking the patient to clench his thumb in the palm of his hand and then the examiner passively pushes the hand into ulnar deviation thus stretching the tendons over the radial styloid process and eliciting pain if tendinitis is present there. In sprain of the first carpal-metacarpal joint, this sign is negative. X-ray films in sprain of the first carpal-metacarpal joint are negative, although similar clinical findings are present when degenerative arthritis occurs at this joint.

Missed Fractures or Dislocations, Multiple

Missed fractures or dislocations in the arm are something that must be guarded against. When a fracture of the shoulder is present, dislocation or fracture of the wrist can also be present and can be easily missed. Furthermore, a dislocation at the proximal end of the elbow at the radio-ulnar joint, for instance, can be missed easily when there is a fracture of the distal end of the ulna. This Monteggia type of fracture dislocation is especially common in children, and there is then a fracture of the shaft towards the distal end of the ulna. If the x-ray films do not include the proximal end of the ulna and radius, a dislocation of the radial ulnar joint can easily be missed.

Dislocations may be missed by not having absolutely accurate anteroposterior and lateral views of the injured extremity. The anteroposterior view may show no dislocation, and the oblique view of an elbow may be of little help. It is absolutely necessary to have an accurate lateral view as well as an absolutely accurate AP view of every injured part.

After an injury to the arm, the entire extremity must be ex-

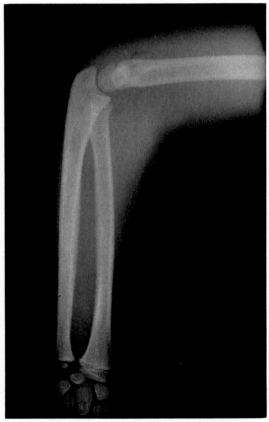

Figure 14A. Lateral view of elbow of a 6-year-old child who fell. Absence of the radiolucent fat pad anterior to the elbow and displacement of the fat pad posterior to the elbow is indicative of a fracture of the distal humerus. A fat pad is radiolucent and this is the "fat pad sign."

amined for other injuries since the patient may not be aware of excessive pain elsewhere in his concentration upon the painful arm.

Acromioclavicular Dislocation

Acromioclavicular dislocation is an injury that is missed especially in the severely injured patient. A patient who has fractures of his legs or has abdominal injury is examined only while he or she is lying down. The dislocation of the clavicle on the cromion reduces itself spontaneously when the patient is lying down. It is

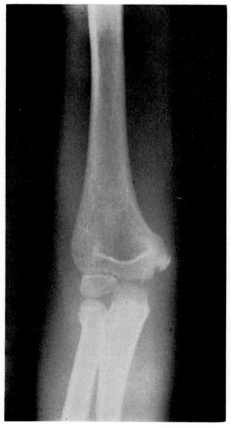

Figure 14B. AP film of the same elbow on thorough examination reveals a faint transverse transcondylar fracture line.

only when the patient has recovered from his more serious injuries and starts sitting up that the monstrous-looking clavicle pops up. Even in the severely injured patient it is possible to examine the patient when the shock has subsided to determine the presence of tenderness in the acromioclavicular area. If the patient cannot be made to sit up to see if any deformity is present and to take an x-ray film in the sitting or standing position preferably, traction on the hand distally can be made and this will separate the clavicle from the acromion. Both visually and by an x-ray film under the shoulder, the diagnosis can be ascertained. If the patient remains seriously ill, he will continue to lie flat in bed and the dislocation may heal spontaneously.

Fractures of the Elbow and Wrist in Children

Fractures of the elbow region and at times at the wrist in children can be difficult to diagnose. There can be minimal displacement, and in fact the fracture line itself may not be visible. The fat pad sign is quite often helpful. This consists of obliteration of the small radiolucent space anterior or posterior to the distal end of the humerus at the site of the fracture when the fracture is present and is not seen through the bone itself. Occasionally, instead of obliteration of the space for the fat pad, this space is seen but is displaced away from the bone. This sign is caused by the presence of hemorrhagic exudate as a result of the fracture.

Fracture of the Proximal Phalanx of the Finger

Fracture of the base of the proximal phalanx of the finger is overlooked often because the fracture site is hidden by the other fingers in the lateral view. Although the fracture itself may be seen in the AP view of the x-ray film, the lateral view hides angular displacement of considerable significance. If the fracture of the proximal phalanx of the finger is to be correctly diagnosed, in addition to the usual views the injured finger must be separated from the others to obtain a satisfactory lateral view, and oblique views may be made. Otherwise the fracture will heal with angulation and not only the involved finger will be limited and painful, but the other fingers will be limited also because of the tethering action of the extensor and other tendons of the fingers.

HYPERPARATHYROIDISM

Hyperparathyroidism is a disease that is frequently overlooked. The disease occurs more frequently in females and is present in the third to the fifth decades of life. Symptoms include weakness and polyuria. Not all patients with hyperparathyroidism have bone disease, however. Bone pain is present with bone involvement. Pathologic fractures and deformities take place, and arthritis also. There may be peptic ulcer and pancreatitis and cerebral disorientation as a result of the increased calcium in the serum. Calcium stones in the kidneys are common.

Radiologically there is subperiosteal bone absorption and diffuse bone atrophy. X-ray films of the mandible reveal resorption of the lamina dura.

Because there is occasionally only one bone lesion instead of diffuse involvement of the skeleton, it is important to determine blood calcium levels in all bone disease.

Secondary hyperparathyroidism can be present as a result of renal glomerular disease. The alkaline phosphatase level is elevated in hyperparathyroidism. Sclerosis or increased density of bone is occasionally found in renal disease with secondary hyperparathyroidism. Interestingly enough, occasionally even in primary hyperparathyroidism but exceedingly rarely there is sclerosis of some of the bones.

CRETINISM OR CHILDHOOD HYPOTHYROIDISM

Cretinism or childhood hypothyroidism is another disease that is frequently not diagnosed first. It is confused with coxa plana or multiple epiphyseal dysplasia. It is of course extremely important to make the diagnosis early so that proper treatment with

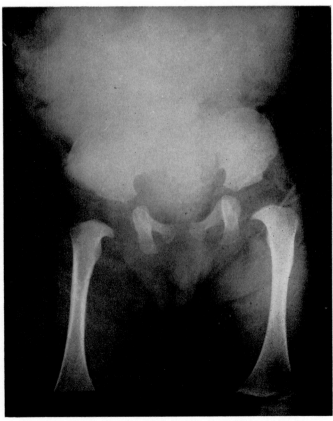

Figure 15A. Cretinism. Note the absence of the capital femoral epiphysis in this 9-year-old female. Early diagnosis is important.

thyroid hormone be given to avoid permanent disability. In cretinism, there is delayed appearance and delayed fusion of all the epiphyses. There may be stippling of the epiphyses as well. In the vertebral column there is kyphosis and flattening of the bodies with increase in width of the intervertebral spaces. There may be some wedging of vertebral bodies. Clinically, the child shows some defective mentality.

The diagnosis is ascertained by appropriate laboratory tests and by the response to thyroid medication.

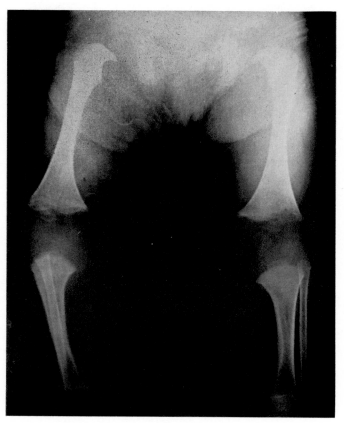

Figure 15B. Same patient. Note the delayed development of the distal femoral and proximal tibial epiphyses.

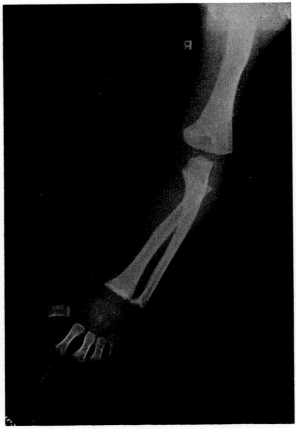

Figure 15C.   Films of the hand show marked retardation of development of the epiphyses in this 9-year-old girl with hypothyroidism.

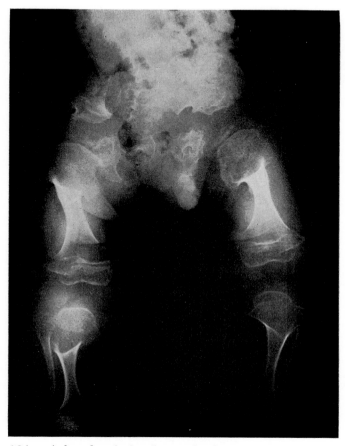

Figure 16A. Achondroplasia, hyperplastic type, in a 14-month-old child. Note the shortening of the femora. The fibulae are longer than normal in comparison with the tibiae. It is important to separate and delineate the many types of dwarfism if any progress in understanding them can be made.

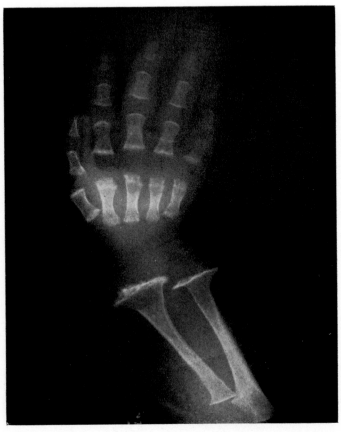

Figure 16B. Forearm and hand in child with achondroplasia. The metaphyses are splayed and broadened. Shortening of the bones is also present.

DEVELOPMENTAL ABNORMALITIES

Dysplasia Epiphysealis Multiplex

This affection is of some practical importance because it is hereditary and because it is easily confused with ordinary degenerative arthritis of the joints. It affects many of the joints of the body, chiefly the hips, knees, and ankles. Occasionally the vertebrae

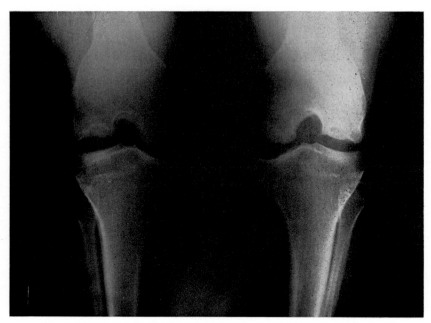

Figure 17. Multiple epiphyseal dysplasia (Fairbanks' disease). This condition is familial and the patient whose knees are shown has a sister with a similar affection. There is bilateral symmetrical irregularity of the epiphyses. The ossification centers demonstrate delayed growth. These irregularitis of the epiphyses occur at many of the joints. Later in life the joints have the appearance of widespread degenerative arthritis.

are involved with irregular vertebral bodies such as hemivertebra or anterior wedging.

The x-ray picture is one of irregularity and at times mottling of the epiphyses. There may be some metaphyseal irregularity at times also. Pain and stiffness of the hips and knees are common complaints in the early onset of degenerative arthritis. There are no abnormalities as far as the sedimentation rate, calcium, phosphorus, and so forth are concerned. The disease is confused with such conditions as cretinism, dysplasia epiphysealis punctata, and generalized osteoarthritis.

Dysplasia Epiphysealis Hemimelica

Dysplasia epiphysealis hemimelica (Trevor's disease) is also of clinical importance because of the marked tendency of the tumors that form to recur after they are excised. The lesion is an osteocartilaginous exostosis limited to one half of an epiphysis. It grows from the cartilaginous articular cartilage. As the articular, or epiarticular exostosis, as Luck calls it, grows, it interferes with motion of the joint and pain develops as well. There is often diminished growth as well as varus or valgus deformity. The most frequent sites of involvement are the talus, the distal femur, and the distal tibia.

It is unknown for the tumor to become malignant, but recurrence of the growth is common and repeated excision is necessary therefore until growth of the patient is complete.

TENDON RUPTURES

Ruptures of tendons are missed occasionally. The experienced orthopedist or any other type of physician who treats patients who have been injured is well aware of the possibility of a ruptured tendon in many areas of the body when the patient says that he has been injured in any way.

Probably the tendon rupture that is most commonly overlooked is that of the tendo Achillis. The patient may have an insignificant injury, or the stress on the leg may be quite great, as in playing tennis. He will complain of pain in his ankle or foot and will have some limp. A conscientious physician will take x-ray films, which will reveal no bone injury. If, however, the physician views the films carefully, he may see distortion of the soft tissue shadow of the tendo Achillis in the lateral view of the ankle. The normal outline of the tendo Achillis is obscured by the hemorrhage that is present when the tendon is ruptured. What is more important is the clinical examination of the patient. There will be some tenderness in the region of the heel cord and a hiatus will be felt there. Unfortunately, if the patient is not examined early, all that may be palpated is tenderness and swelling inasmuch as the disruption of the tendon becomes hidden by the swelling and hemorrhage. The patient is asked to stand on the toes of the involved foot, raising himself up there without the aid of the normal foot. If he is unable to do this, to raise his weight from the floor on the toes of the injured leg, the tendo Achillis is almost certainly ruptured. If the much more innocuous injury of partial gastrocnemius muscle fiber rupture or rupture of the plantaris tendon is present, there will be pain with this maneuver but the patient will be able to rise up on his toes without any real difficulty.

It is of the utmost importance to distinguish between injury consisting of a torn plantaris tendon or gastrocnemius muscle fibers compared with the disabling rupture of the tendo Achillis.

The latter injury must be treated or permanent weakness of the leg will be present, whereas the former conditions, namely gastrocnemius muscle tears or plantaris tendon rupture, will heal without any treatment.

Other tendons of the foot—the anterior tibial, posterior tibial, and flexor hallucis—may all be ruptured. Sometimes a tiny penetrating wound by a piece of glass or some other sharp instrument may cut the tendon, and yet the laceration may be so trivial as to be overlooked. The insertion of the posterior tibial tendon is occasionally nicked and then the patient will develop progressive valgus deformity if the laceration is missed and not repaired. When the patient complains of pain or weakness of a foot or leg, strength of all the muscles of the ankle and foot should be examined. This will take only several moments to do and is well worthwhile.

In the region of the knee, the quadriceps tendon or the patellar ligament, where it attaches from the patella to the tibial tubercle, can be ruptured and these lesions can be overlooked. It is important, therefore, that after any knee injury the strength of the quadriceps mechanism be examined by asking the patient to keep the knee extended against the resistance of the examiner's arm. The x-ray films that would be taken may also help in a small way to disclose the disruption of the soft tissue shadow of these tendons.

In the hip area, avulsion ruptures of the rectus tendon from the ilium are not too uncommon an injury, and although this particular tendon rupture usually requires no sugical treatment, it is helpful to make the diagnosis so that a more serious lesion is not diagnosed. A hiatus will be felt at the site of origin of the rectus muscle at the anterior aspect of the ilium, and the abnormal bulging of the rectus muscle in the thigh area will be seen when the patient is asked to keep his knee straight against resistance.

Hamstring tendon ruptures are fairly common and need no specific treatment usually, but the avulsed tendon will form a lump. When one is unaware of the possibility of this condition, it may be misdiagnosed as a tumor and unnecessary surgical exploration will therefore be done.

In the abdomen, rupture of the rectus abdominis is commonly misdiagnosed as an intraperitoneal lesion. The tenderness superficially of the muscle and the pain on contracture of the abdominal wall muscles, as well as the absence of any systemic signs of disease, will lead the examiner to the correct diagnosis.

In the arm, the common rupture of the long head of the biceps muscle is found only by asking the patient to flex the elbow against the resistance of the examiner's arm. The tenderness in the region of the biceptial groove in the upper humerus, plus the abnormal bulging of the biceps in the mid third of the upper arm, will then be seen. In the fat person, this bulging must be searched for because it will not be obvious.

Rupture of the supraspinatus tendon is often a difficult type of diagnosis to make. It can take place without any significant injury in the elderly or even middle-aged person. In addition to pain in the shoulder area, there should be noticeable weakness of abduction against the resistance of the examiner's arm. This diagnosis, ruptured supraspinatus tendon, can be verified by arthrography of the shoulder joint.

Ruptures of the triceps tendon can occur as well as of other muscles of the arm and forearm. Weakness of elbow extension and the presence of a gap in the tendon help in arriving at the correct diagnosis.

Ruptures of the flexor or extensor tendons of the fingers occur and are missed once in a while. If there is a disease of the wrist or hand, such as rheumatoid arthritis, such ruptures are much more common, and in those instances the ruptures usually occur in the wrist area. In other instances, the rupture more commonly occurs at the distal insertion of the tendon at the distal phalanx. Rupture of the flexor profundus tendon can occur after some strain, and if one is not observant it will not be seen. The strength of the flexor tendons should be tested after any injury of the finger, and this applies as well to the extensor tendon. Trick movements by the lumbrical muscles can make the fingers move in the presence of a ruptured long tendon. There will, however, be absent flexon on extension of the tip of the finger. To test for isolated rupture of the flexor sublimus tendon, hold all the other three fingers extended while the patient tries to flex the involved finger. By doing this, the flexor profundus action is prevented and if the finger flexes at the proximal interphalangeal joint, then the sublimus tendon is intact.

SPRAIN OF THE COSTOCHONDRAL JUNCTION

This affection is a peculiar and ill-defined one. If it occurs in the upper rib area near the sternum, it has been called Tzieze's syndrome and is often confused with angina pectoris.

The diagnosis is made by exclusion. Disease of the ribs and bone is excluded by x-ray films revealing no abnormality, and intrathoracic disease is excluded by thorough evaluation of the heart and lungs.

With costochondral sprain, there is tenderness at the junction at the rib and costal cartilage, or between the costal cartilage and the sternum. If this point tenderness is present and other diseases as noted above have been excluded, the diagnosis of costochondral sprain can be made and the patient reassured that there is no severe disease present. He will get well spontaneously.

IMPINGEMENT OF THE RIB CAGE ON THE ILIUM

In the adult patient with severe scoliosis or kyphosis, the rib cage can touch and rub on the superior portion of the ilium. This will cause pain, and the patient will be fearful because he does not understand the source of the pain. Of course, the patient who has severe deformity of the dorsal spine, such as kyphosis or scoliosis, can also have all types of abdominal disease that could mimic this condition. Indeed, he is usually labeled as having some intra-abdominal condition such as colitis or gastritis. It goes without saying that a complete examination of the abdominal viscera should be done to exclude these diseases. If then the physician is left with a patient who has tenderness at the distal end of the rib cage and he finds that the rib cage does touch the iliac crest of the pelvis, he can make the diagnosis of impingement of the rib cage. The diagnosis may be verified by injecting the tender area with a dilute solution of Xylocaine. Pain should be relieved for at least an hour. Care must be taken to have the injection superficial in order to prevent perforation of the lung or peritoneum.

THE SEVERELY INJURED PATIENT

Fat embolism is to be suspected in every severely injured patient. The diagnosis is usually not made until late in the disease. Every patient who sustains a fracture of a long bone should be suspected of having fat embolism if he becomes delirious. The signs of fat embolism are tachycardia, fever, dyspnea and rapidly developing anemia. The tell-tale petechia on the chest or abdomen are almost pathognomonic of fat embolism. The suspected patient should have an examination of urine for fat and lipase studies of the blood will also be helpful. Many other conditions such as pulmonary atelectasis, thrombophlebitis with pulmonary embolism, subdural hematomas of the brain will cause signs and symptoms similar to those of fat embolism. The severely injured patient must be monitored carefully. Such things as central venous pressure determinations, blood CO_2 and O_2 determinations are necessary.

The help of a competent internist or general surgeon is usually mandatory. In the severely injured patient, repeated examinations must be made of the entire body to make sure that injuries elsewhere are not overlooked. Fractures of the mandible, fractures of the hip, fractures of the spine, are easy to miss in the patient that has had a severe injury elsewhere. Arterial injuries as well as nerve injuries must be looked for repeatedly.

Intra-abdominal and intra-thoracic injuries of all types may be present and the orthopedist must rely on the internist or general surgeon for such injuries but nevertheless he should not depend completely on his colleagues.

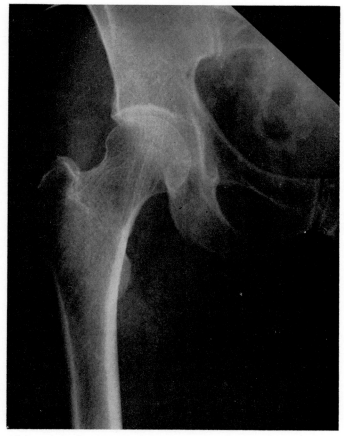

Figure 18A.   AP view of the femur after an injury. No fracture seen.

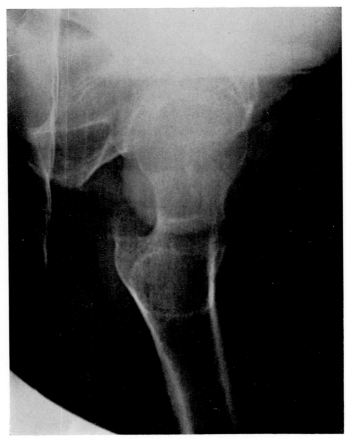

Figure 18B. Lateral view is also negative.

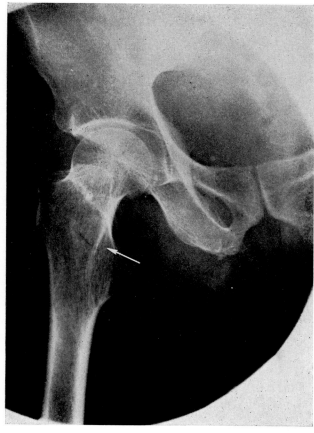

Figure 18C. Only in an oblique view is a fracture line through the trochanteric area seen. The importance of multiple views in a suspected fracture is thus emphasized.

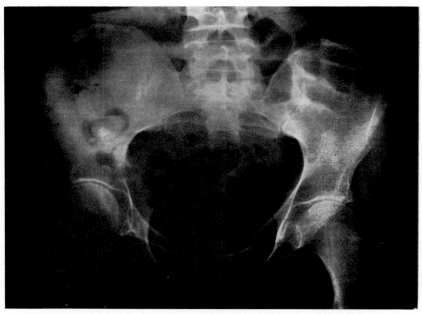

Figure 19A. The film of the femoral neck after a fall reveals no fracture.

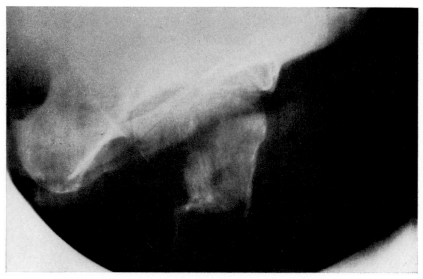

Figure 19B.   Lateral view also reveals no fracture.

Difficult Orthopedic Diagnosis

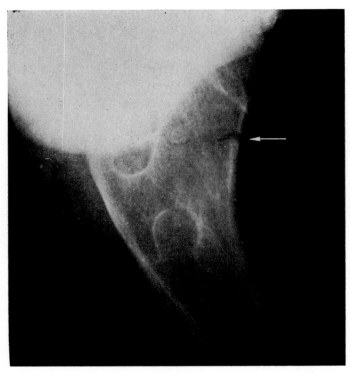

Figure 19C. Because of continued pain a film was made one week later showing a fracture of the neck of the femur. It is important to re–x-ray hips that are painful after any injury.

POLYMYALGIA RHEUMATICA

This condition of elderly people is characterized by very painful joints, more often in the upper extremities such as the shoulder. The patient, an elderly or middle-aged woman or man, complains of inordinate pain in the shoulders or the leg. The pain is ill-defined. There is pain on any attempt to move the extremities, especially the arm. The diffuse tenderness around the shoulder joint area may simulate tendinitis and bursitis. There is no effusion in the joint. The patient is anxious, fatigues easily, and sleeps poorly. Low grade fever is often present. The sedimentation rate is almost universally elevated. There may be accompanying giant cell arteritis, especially of the temporal arteries.

The diagnosis is readily missed, and a diagnosis of neurosis or of degenerative arthritis or even of rheumatoid arthritis is made instead of the correct one of polymyalgia rheumatica.

The diagnosis is aided by the prompt response to corticosteroid therapy.

In this connection the polymyositis with or without a skin rash accompanying malignancies should be remembered.

THORACIC DISC PROTRUSION

This is a difficult diagnosis to make. The patient will experience vague pain usually in the rib areas. There may be some vague pains in both legs as a result of this type of protrusion in the thoracic spine. Once in a while there is evidence of long tract signs involving the legs. In other words, there may be hyperactive reflexes of slight degree or the reflexes may be unequal. Babinski reflexes may also be present in one or both legs.

There is often hypesthesia to touch and pain prick of one thoracic nerve root. Tenderness is present over a spinous process of the involved disc and there is pain usually with hyperextension of the dorsal spine.

The x-ray films will usually show either narrowing of the disc space or calcification of the disc space. A pantopaque myelogram will make the diagnosis certain.

CAT SCRATCH DISEASE

A disease usually missed is that of lymphadenitis caused by cat scratch virus. There is usually a mass in one of the lymph nodes. This can be easily mistaken for a sarcoma. The mass is usually slightly tender and nonfluctuant but at times may be fluctuant. Low grade fever may be present and the sedimentation rate is usually slightly elevated.

The diagnosis is ascertained by injecting .1 ml of cat scratch antigen interdermally. Induration of the injected area occurs within one or two days.

HERPES ZOSTER

This may occur over one or more dermatomes. The first symptom is pain. The patient is usually elderly or middle-aged but occasionally can be quite young. Pain varies in degree but is usually fairly severe and can be excruciating. After the pain is present, there is hyperesthesia corresponding to the distribution of the dermatome. There may be a low grade fever early in the disease. The diagnosis is often missed because during the first week or so there are no manifestations of the disease other than pain. The joints of the involved area move normally and motion does not make the pain worse. X-ray films reveal no abnormality of the associated bony structure.

The burning pain is somewhat characteristic, but it is only when the rash occurs that the diagnosis becomes evident. The rash is a vesicular one leaving crusted elevations. If for some reason the rash is not seen, postherpetic neuralgia may be present when the rash clears and this in itself can be very painful.

INDEX